Rockhaven
SANITARIUM

Rockhaven
SANITARIUM

The Legacy of Agnes Richards

Elisa Jordan

THE
History
PRESS

Published by The History Press
Charleston, SC
www.historypress.com

All images courtesy of the Friends of Rockhaven unless otherwise noted.

First published 2018

Manufactured in the United States

ISBN 9781467138796

Library of Congress Control Number: 2018945794

Notice: The information in this book is true and complete to the best of our knowledge. It is offered without guarantee on the part of the author or The History Press. The author and The History Press disclaim all liability in connection with the use of this book.

This book is dedicated to Agnes Richards, Patricia Traviss and the entire staff, employees and residents who made Rockhaven special. Thanks to their devotion and kindness, they turned Rockhaven into a safe place for women to heal in safety and with dignity. In the process, they made history with a progressive approach to mental health, women's wellness and career opportunities for women. Gladys Monroe Baker deserves a mention because it was her story that originally brought me to Rockhaven. Without her, this book would never have happened. I would also like to dedicate this book to the Friends of Rockhaven, the next generation of dedicated people working to preserve this landmark for the future.

Contents

Acknowledgements

This book wouldn't be possible without the gracious help of the Friends of Rockhaven. This dedicated nonprofit group has single-handedly worked to preserve the property, legacy and future of Rockhaven Sanitarium. Their tireless efforts were an inspiration to me during the entire process of researching and writing this book. I'd like to specifically thank Joanna Linkchorst and Mike Lawler for granting me access to their Rockhaven files, photos and research materials. They not only permitted me to go through the Rockhaven archives but also patiently answered questions, read drafts and were exceptionally supportive of me during the writing process. Thanks to my editor at The History Press, Laurie Krill, who guided me through the publishing process and helped me turn an idea into an actual book. She has been a rock through the entire experience. Thanks to Eve Adamson Minkler, my friend and fellow writer, whose advice I always take. Scott Fortner, Jackie Craig and April VeVea were enormously helpful with research. My friend Lynn Garrett looked at photos for me and helped give her expert advice. My cousin John Garside scanned photos for me. Thanks to my parents, Gene and Victoria Jordan, who have long supported my love of (and obsession with) literature, history and education. Our family road trips exploring local landmarks have had an enormous influence on me. And finally, thank you to my friends and family who have supported me and all my crazy ideas over the years. I am deeply humbled and grateful.

Introduction

My Rockhaven journey actually begins years ago while researching Marilyn Monroe. I had read about her mother Gladys's history of mental illness and hospitalization at a private sanitarium named Rockhaven. It was at Rockhaven that Gladys came to live as soon as Marilyn's finances allowed. I never expected to actually see inside Rockhaven's gates, but I immediately signed up when I saw that tours were offered of the now-historic landmark. That was May 2014, and little did I know that my life was about to change when I stepped foot onto the grounds.

As soon as I laid eyes on Rockhaven, it became clear that it was a place like no other. Although there was some peeling paint and withered flower beds, it still exuded a sense of tranquility. Seeing the property in person and learning of the facility's progressive practices and importance to women's history brought to life a world I didn't know existed. I had to know more.

Agnes Richards was a German immigrant and single mother trying to earn a living to support her young son. With limited career options available to her, she worked her way through nursing school and found employment in state-funded mental hospitals. To Agnes, working in institutions became much more than just a job. She cared about her patients and sought to improve hospital conditions. She also provided jobs to women who, like her, found few options when it came to work opportunities.

Introduction

My goal with this book is to document the story of Rockhaven from its inception through the glory days up to the present. That Agnes Richards founded a private sanitarium catering to female patients and employing a mostly female staff decades before the women's movement is itself an accomplishment. That it was so successful adds an extra element.

Chapter 1

A Short History
of the Crescenta Valley

The Crescenta Valley is a suburban community nestled among the San Gabriel Mountains to the northeast and the Verdugo Mountains and San Rafael Hills to the southwest. The San Gabriel Valley lies to La Crescenta's southeast and the San Fernando Valley to the northwest. Though it is now a fairly typical suburb of Los Angeles, the area's history dates back thousands of years to a thriving Native American community. The Tongva (also called Gabrieleño) lived peacefully in the valley until the late 1700s.

European explorers first noticed what is present-day California in the 1500s, with the Spanish empire claiming the land in 1542. Sebastian Vizcaino later mapped the region for New Spain in 1602, though the Crown paid little attention to the area or its native inhabitants for generations. During this time, California's native population was culturally and linguistically diverse, with more than seventy Native American groups settled in California. Estimates for the native population range from 100,000 to 300,000 depending on the source, but the one thing that is certain is the region was thriving. Although rich with resources, the land was difficult to access for outsiders, so Spain largely left California alone.

Life in California began to change under the rule of Charles III. With news making its way back to Spain of Russian fur traders in the remote colony, Charles decided to gain control of the region. In 1769, the first California mission was established. From that moment on, settlers and missionaries began making their way to the once largely ignored colony. Between 1769 and 1833, twenty-one missions would eventually line what is now the state of California. It was also the beginning of the genocide of native peoples in the region.

In 1784, the Spanish Crown granted 36,402 acres of land to Jose Maria Verdugo, a soldier who served at the San Gabriel Mission. The land grant bordered what is now the Arroyo Seco and Los Angeles River and included the modern-day Crescenta Valley, Glendale and parts of Burbank and the Verdugo Mountains, which were named in Verdugo's honor. Corporal Verdugo retired from the army in 1798 and became a full-time rancher on his property, Rancho San Rafael. The rancho was inherited by Verdugo's children after his death in 1831, but his heirs didn't hang onto the property for as long as their father. The land survived the Mexican-American War but didn't last much longer than that.

By the late 1800s, the area was attracting health seekers and tourists from other parts of the United States. The warm, dry climate was ideal for those in need of lung ailment recovery and respite from cold, wet winters.

One of those people in search of a better, healthier climate was Dr. Benjamin Briggs. After losing his first wife, Abigail, to tuberculosis, Dr. Briggs began searching for ways to help other patients with lung ailments. Briggs remarried, to Abigail's sister Caroline, and began searching for the ideal place to open his treatment facility.

Briggs's own health was poor. It was likely that Briggs had tuberculosis like his first wife; he also had a gunshot wound that never quite healed correctly. Either way, his interest in health and lung ailments led to a search for the perfect property, which eventually brought him to present-day Crescenta Valley. Once he discovered the area, Briggs knew he had found his dream location. In 1881, he set about purchasing a large section of land, first a homestead and then expanding to include the valley. His property stretched from Pickens Canyon to Tujunga.

It was Briggs who named the valley Crescenta. There are two stories as to how he came up with the name. One says that when Briggs looked out his window, he could make out three crescents in the landscape. The other story says that a crescent shape appears in the way the land forms around the valley. Because *crescenta* is not a Spanish word, it's likely that Briggs made up the word, inspired by a crescent shape of some sort in the surrounding landscape. It is generally believed that the post office added the La to Crescenta to distinguish it from Northern California's Crescent City.

Briggs's idea of making the Crescenta Valley a destination for those suffering with lung ailments proved to be a good one, and other sanitariums

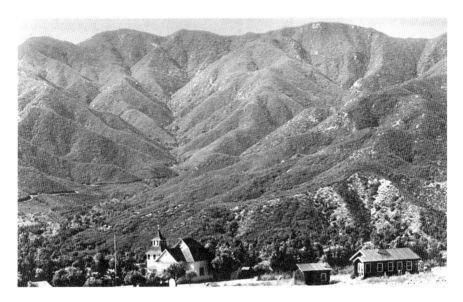

The area near the Verdugo Mountains dates back thousands of years to when it was home to thriving Native American communities until the late 1700s. In the 1800s, the region's warm, dry climate made it ideal for those seeking treatment for lung ailments. *Courtesy of the Glendale Public Library.*

soon followed in the valley. Although lung disease was the original focus of health seekers in the area, sanitariums for mental health also established themselves in the valley. Some of the other well-known sanitariums that followed Briggs's lead include Kimball Sanitarium, where actress Frances Farmer would one day be placed, and Rockhaven, the sanitarium for women.

Briggs proved to be a pioneer not just of the sanitarium industry in Crescenta but of the city as well. He established a city center and subdivided his surrounding land into ten-acre lots. But the area's success had consequences on the once-clean air. The climate that had once attracted tourists and health seekers to the rural area began to change. As the decades wore on, the population grew, increasing the number of cars filling the streets. Smog and pollution hung in the air, and because La Crescenta is a valley, much of that putrid air was trapped by the surrounding hills, no longer making the area ideal for health seekers and those with lung ailments.

By the 1960s, the area had become a fairly standard post–World War II suburb of Los Angeles. The suburbanization of the area continued with the opening of the Foothill Freeway (210) in 1972, the Glendale Freeway (2) opening and Interstate 5 in 1978.

This was the ever-changing background in which Agnes Richards set up Rockhaven, which not only made history as a women's facility but was also the very last of the sanitariums in the area to close. The business she so lovingly set up survived the changes of the mental health industry; it also survived all the changes happening in and around the valley.

Chapter 2

Agnes Richards, the Woman Who Founded Rockhaven

O ne of the most remarkable aspects of Rockhaven Sanitarium is that it was opened and run *by* women and *for* women before the women's movement. Agnes Richards was a woman and health professional decades ahead of her time. When she opened Rockhaven in 1923, women had only won the right to vote in the United States just three years before. It was a time when most women didn't attend college, let alone open a business or especially a sanitarium. Agnes's unique approach to life and her ability to accomplish the seemingly impossible stemmed from her ability to create and invent. That includes not just Rockhaven but herself as well.

When Agnes was older, the official biography she liked to share about herself was that she was born in the American Midwest and educated in Germany during her youth. The years of her birth mysteriously changed, depending on the documentation in question. In fact, she was born Agnes Lepinski in Germany on February 16, 1881. The family's origins were humble, and like many people in the late 1800s, they dreamed of a better life in the United States.

Agnes's father, August, arrived ahead of the others on June 8, 1893, aboard a ship called the *Dresden*. The rest of the Lepinskis, which included his wife, Anna, and children (Agnes, another daughter and two sons) arrived a few months later on the *Darmstadt* on September 19. It's not known why August traveled ahead of his family, but the most likely explanation is that he established himself in America first before sending for the rest of the family.

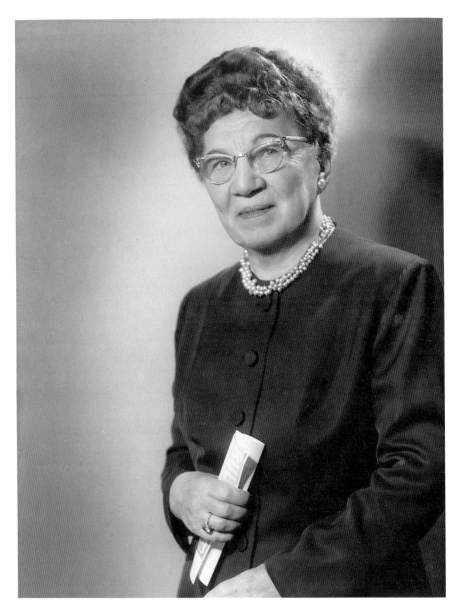

Agnes Richards founded Rockhaven Sanitarium in 1923, decades before the women's movement. She started off as a German immigrant who endured young widowhood, single motherhood, working through nursing school, working in mental hospitals and going on to become a successful entrepreneur.

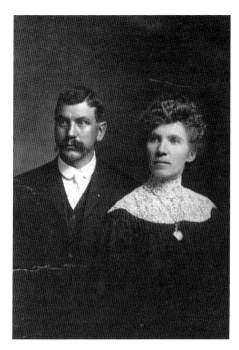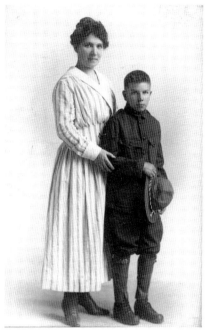

Left: Agnes Lepinski married her first husband, David Traviss, on August 3, 1904. The marriage ended just a year and a half later when David was struck and killed by a motor vehicle in January 1906. His death meant Agnes suddenly found herself alone with an infant son to support.

Right: Agnes and her young son, Clarence Walter Traviss.

A new country allowed the family to reinvent themselves once in the United States. That desire for reinvention informed Agnes for the rest of her life, not just in the stories she told about herself but also in the life she actually led. She showed a talent for bettering herself, updating her skill sets and moving to new locations when necessary.

The Lepinskis settled in the township of Denver, Nebraska, where August and Agnes, as the oldest child, supported the family as day laborers, according to the 1900 census. But Agnes wouldn't remain a day laborer forever. On August 3, 1904, records show she married David Traviss in Chicago. Her marriage to David was short-lived, as he was struck by a car and killed on January 16, 1906, in Chicago at the age of thirty-seven.

Although they had been married just a year and a half, they produced a son, Clarence Walter Traviss, born in July 1905. With the death of her husband, Agnes was in need of a job to support herself and her infant son.

Perhaps to regroup and be closer to her family, Agnes left Chicago and returned to Nebraska, where she took a job as a "servant" at the Nebraska State Hospital for the Insane. It was likely her first experience working in an asylum, which was housed in an imposing brick facility. It was here that she began her journey into the world of mental healthcare, and as the years progressed, she witnessed how different hospitals treated their patients. Through her observations, she noted what helped, what made things worse, what was abusive and myriad other details that others frequently overlooked or ignored.

Agnes was clearly attentive and ambitious, as she worked her way up to an attendant position and found herself employed at Independence State Hospital in Iowa. Like the hospital in Nebraska, it was a state-funded facility that housed the insane. Also like Nebraska State Hospital, the circa 1870s building gave the appearance of a foreboding structure. Both hospitals looked intimidating when one pulled up in front with a loved one who was about to walk through the doors.

Independence State Hospital proved to be a turning point for Agnes. As she continued to learn about the mental health industry on the frontlines, she met another attendant named James Richards, whom she married on April 10, 1917. Now enjoying more financial security, instead of quitting and becoming a traditional wife, Agnes used the opportunity to expand her education and career.

When the United States entered World War I, Agnes went where she believed she could do the most good. She volunteered for the Red Cross and was assigned to active duty at Camp Dodge, a 3,500-acre military camp near Des Moines. Camp Dodge served as a training facility for infantry and a demobilization center for soldiers returning home. It was also home to officers and support personnel, of whom Agnes was one. The base included housing, an auditorium, an Information Bureau, a YMCA, a YWCA, a hospital and a Red Cross building.

Patient life on the base would have differed vastly from an asylum. Combat veterans would have been returning from war with shell shock (now called PTSD), which would have expanded what she was already used to. She also received additional training in injuries, disfigurements and illnesses.

Although it's not certain, it may be because of the war (and later World War II) that Agnes hid her German birth. Anti-German sentiment was strong in the United States at the time, so it's not unreasonable that she might want to present herself as born on American soil. Claiming she was educated in Germany during her youth would explain how she could speak both

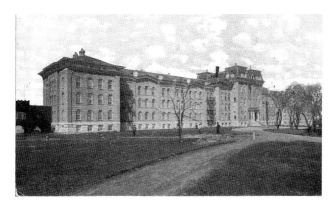

Agnes worked at Nebraska State Hospital for the Insane during her early years in the mental healthcare industry. The architecture of the structure was fairly typical for its time: large, imposing and enclosed. Agnes observed that such buildings looked intimidating and could frighten patients and make their relatives feel uncomfortable during visits. *Author's collection.*

German and English without an accent in either language. It would also give her life story an extra panache that her humble beginnings lacked, but there is likely more to her reasoning than just spinning a good story. Records indicate that at least one of her brothers was also hiding his German origins by claiming to have been born in Wisconsin, including in his World War II draft paperwork. Clearly, both brother and sister felt there was a need to falsify their birthplace.

To continue building on her experience, Agnes enrolled in a program at Cook County Hospital to receive her RN degree, which she eventually earned in 1922. After the war, she and her husband left the Midwest for good and moved to California, where she once again found herself working for asylums. For the next few years, Agnes worked for two asylums in Southern California. The first was Patton State Hospital in San Bernardino in 1920, which was followed by Los Angeles General Hospital in 1922. Like the asylums she had worked for in the Midwest, these were government-run hospitals. According to records, her husband, James Richards, also worked at Patton. During this time, Agnes worked as a head nurse, which brought with it a higher level of skills for practicing various aspects of healthcare. She also possessed experience in leadership, management and administration.

After working as a nurse in asylums in the late 1910s and early 1920s, Agnes had some fairly astute assessments of American psychiatric care. The reasons for admission ranged from serious mental illness to the ridiculous, such as masturbation, epilepsy, grief, depression, paralysis, head injuries, poverty, addiction and more. What was worse was the treatment many patients received while hospitalized.

Often there was no treatment at all; in retrospect, many health conditions were made worse by the poor living conditions. Hospitals of yesterday can't be held responsible for treatments that did not yet exist. However, many asylums subjected their patients to inhumane environments for any era. Conditions were vastly improving during the turn of the twentieth century, thanks in large part to an exposé by undercover reporter Nellie Bly, who wrote about atrocities she witnessed while living as a "patient" in an asylum. But even after Bly's exposé, patients were still often poorly fed or starved; sometimes they were confined like prison inmates. In many cases, they were forced to work against their will or were victims of physical violence, either by overzealous staff or other patients.

Agnes also noticed that asylums held additional risks for women, who were exceptionally vulnerable to institutionalization. Because women had significantly fewer rights than men, they were susceptible to male family members admitting them against their will. It wasn't unheard of for husbands to declare their wives insane for postpartum depression, menopause or "noncompliance." In this regard, institutionalization would have been a viable option for some men to avoid divorce during a time when it was a social taboo.

Even for sane women subjected to asylum life, their stability would eventually deteriorate into ill mental health at some point, in one way or another. The women who did have mental illnesses had little to no chance of improving their conditions due to poor physical and mental treatment. Further, women in these hospitals experienced the threat of danger from male employees, attendants or other inmates. Women were, unfortunately, vulnerable to sexual abuse at the hands of those entrusted to care for them or their fellow patients. Because they had no recourse, no rights or were physically or mentally impaired, they were easy prey for predators.

Agnes was appalled at institutional conditions and decided she had seen enough. She knew she could do better. She dreamed of providing a safe, healing environment for women in need of mental healthcare and rest. Fortunately for her, she was in the right place at the right time. Psychiatric care was about to experience a progressive renaissance, and California was at the head of that movement.

She set her eyes on the Crescenta Valley, which was already the location of several sanitariums. The clean, dry air and open land made it the ideal location for hospitals. Agnes's first step in opening her sanitarium was

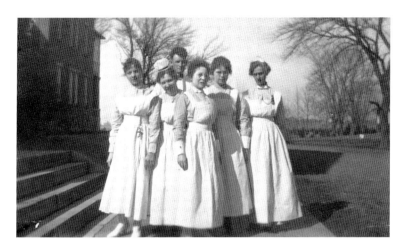

Agnes Richards, *center*, as a young nurse.

renting a stone house that had once been a family home. The choice of architecture was no accident. The large, hulking buildings she had previously worked in could appear intimidating and feel impersonal. Her sanitarium would feel like a real home and a haven from the outside world. Taking a cue from the house's stone exterior and the intention of her business, she christened the property Rockhaven.

Agnes Richards opened Rockhaven Sanitarium in January 1923 with six patients living in the stone house. From the first day, Rockhaven distinguished itself from other sanitariums. Agnes increased safety precautions by hiring a female-only staff. Doctors in this era were men, but anyone who had daily contact with the patients—nurses, attendants and staff—was a woman. It was a decision that not only created an extra measure of security for patients but also provided jobs during an era when it was tougher for women to have careers.

When it came to the patients themselves, Agnes had watched what helped people get well and what caused them further harm. Instead of confinement, for instance, she decided Rockhaven's patients would have access to a yard where they could breathe in fresh air, sit in the sun and enjoy the gardens. Employees took care of Rockhaven's maintenance so there was no need to force patients into hard labor around the property. To keep patients' minds active, Agnes supplied projects and crafts. On special occasions, outings such as lunch were planned so the women could safely experience life outside the sanitarium while still under supervision. In the best-case scenario, it helped

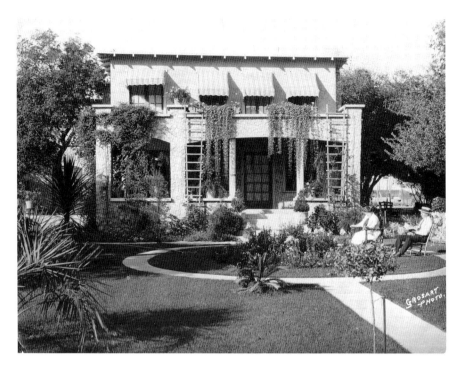

Rockhaven opened in 1923 with just six patients. Instead of a hospital, Agnes selected an actual house so her patients would feel "at home" in their surroundings. She also instructed staff to call the women staying at Rockhaven "ladies" or "residents" as a way to make them more comfortable and retain their dignity.

ease the women back into the world. If a woman likely wouldn't live on her own again, she could still experience fun activities on the outside without feeling isolated. All of these policies were a direct result of Agnes observing that when minds were continually working and kept active, people were far less likely to recede into their illnesses.

Employees at Rockhaven were instructed to treat patients with the utmost respect. The patients may have been experiencing nervous disorders, but treating them with dignity would help them get well. This factor was built into every layer of Rockhaven, from treatment down to administrative policies. Because of Agnes's attention to detail, patients were not to be called "patients." The women staying at Rockhaven were called "ladies" or "residents."

Agnes's progressive approach quickly garnered attention, and more residents moved to Rockhaven. Soon, business grew and the campus expanded, all the while maintaining the high standards set by Agnes herself.

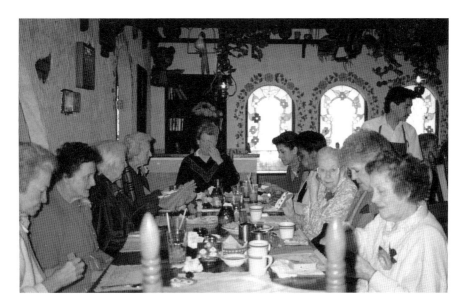

This Valentine's luncheon for the ladies of Rockhaven perfectly demonstrates how the sanitarium liked to keep residents active.

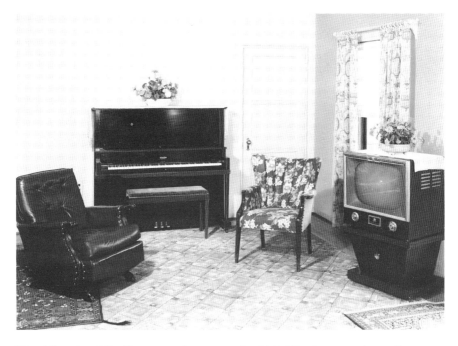

The philosophy of Rockhaven was that women should feel like they are at home. Some of the bungalows even had common areas, or living rooms, that were not unlike a family's house. In this instance, the living room has comfortable chairs, a television set and a piano.

Rockhaven thrived under Agnes's direction, but that didn't mean there weren't challenges to running a successful sanitarium. According to Crescenta Valley historian Mike Lawler, a housing boom hit the area in the 1920s, and the new locals were starting to express resistance to the sanitariums. The valley had long been to home to sanitariums that catered to various conditions, including lung diseases, mental illness and elder care.

Neighbors were understandably resistant to living by facilities catering to infectious diseases, such as tuberculosis. They also didn't want proximity to "insane asylums." The land once considered a haven for those in need of healthcare and rest was now valuable real estate. The community organized and became a remarkably effective political group that attended city council meetings with the specific intention of discussing sanitariums. Neighbors and real estate agents alike attended meetings and even formed a group called the La Crescenta Protective Association, which was made up of prominent residents and businesspeople. Their influence was starting to show itself in city council decisions. Because of their efforts, a sanitarium building permit across from Kimball Sanitarium was denied in 1928.

That same year, the political group turned its attention to Rockhaven when Agnes applied for a permit to expand her business in November 1928. Her request was met with protesters, who testified at city council meetings. Some of their concerns were potentially valid, such as property values and proximity to residential housing (even though the sanitariums were there first). Among their other complaints, however, were absurd accusations. In five years, Rockhaven had grown from housing six women to about thirty. But protesters claimed that Rockhaven was filled with sixty "insane" men and women who had escaped and "ran screaming down the streets of the suburbs at unenjoyable hours of the night." Another resident testified that "wild looking men" were peering through Rockhaven's gates and frightening neighborhood women. (Apparently the protesters forgot to take into account that no men lived on the property.) Other accusations against Rockhaven were that one of the patients had tried to poison the other residents and that Agnes usually worked while drunk. Under pressure from homeowners, the city issued a stop work order on Rockhaven's permit and referred the matter to the county's public welfare committee.

The group's goal had been to ban all sanitariums from the valley, Rockhaven included. Its efforts garnered a lot of success, but in the end, the overzealous behavior and outlandish accusations backfired. Maybe locals didn't like living near sanitariums, but the ridiculous accusations against Rockhaven as a business and Agnes personally exposed the underbelly of the protesters. Agnes wasn't about to stand for false stories about herself or the sanitarium she had painstakingly built. She filed a slander suit against Mrs. Oscar Johnson, one of the locals who had lied about Rockhaven. In her lawsuit, Agnes asked for $100,000. That would be $50,000 actual and $50,000 in damages for statements made at a November 14 meeting in which Mrs. Johnson asserted that Agnes was unfit to run Rockhaven. Mrs. Johnson denied making any such statements, but the case went to trial and Agnes prevailed. She didn't get the $100,000 she initially requested, but she did get $500 in personal damage, $200 in community damage and $100 for penalty. More importantly, her name was cleared publicly, and she was permitted to continue running and expanding Rockhaven.

If the late 1920s had their professional challenges, there were also big changes at home. The 1930 census indicates that Agnes was now divorced and the head of her household. What happened in her marriage is not known, but her personal issues had not interfered with Rockhaven's growth or her fierce protection of it.

Though her first few years in business had not been without turbulence, Agnes had been able to build a successful business and make a positive impact in her community. Starting in the late 1920s, Agnes began serving on the board of directors of the new Crescenta-Canada Bank in Montrose. She was the only woman on the board with some of the community's highest-profile men.

The 1940s were a time of great success for Agnes. For starters, she remarried, and this time, she found her "happily ever after" with a man named Hickman, to whom she was married until he passed away years later. Her professional life similarly thrived. Agnes took over as the director of music for the local Catholic church's Easter Mass. In this role, she reached out to high-end musical talent from Los Angeles for assistance. She appeared to love music, as she was also involved with the Southern California Symphony Association and the California Junior Symphony Orchestra, which she sponsored. She also became active in the La Canada Thursday Club, Los Angeles Breakfast Club, Women's Auxiliary of California Babies' and Children's Hospital, Opera Guild of Southern California, Town and Gown, Women's Committee of Philharmonic, Ballet of Los Angeles and Toastmistress Club. As Rockhaven continued to prosper, she used her business acumen to begin investing in stocks and real estate, which provided her with long-term financial prosperity.

Agnes had built a solid business model, and Rockhaven continued thriving under her leadership. Rockhaven's reputation as a premier sanitarium

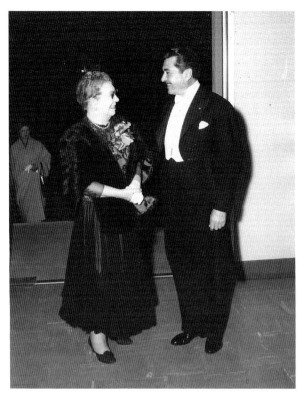

Left: Agnes Richards at the symphony in 1959. Over the years, she became heavily involved in the community and sponsored the Southern California Symphony Association and the California Junior Symphony Orchestra.

Below: Rockhaven built a reputation as one of the finest sanitariums in Southern California. Its brochures emphasized the respect residents received during their stay.

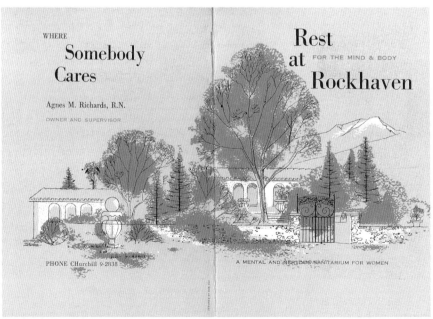

exclusively for women was known throughout the region. And because of its proximity to Los Angeles and Hollywood, Rockhaven attracted prominent women, including from the entertainment industry. At Rockhaven, they were assured the finest care and privacy.

It wasn't just the movie star residents who got star treatment. All women were afforded superior treatment. In addition to all the amenities, field trips and activities, Agnes herself personally connected with the residents, bringing them See's Candies and playing bridge with them. The nurses also benefited from Agnes's personal attention and generosity. She was known to occasionally take nurses to furriers for Christmas to gift them with luxurious furs for jobs well done.

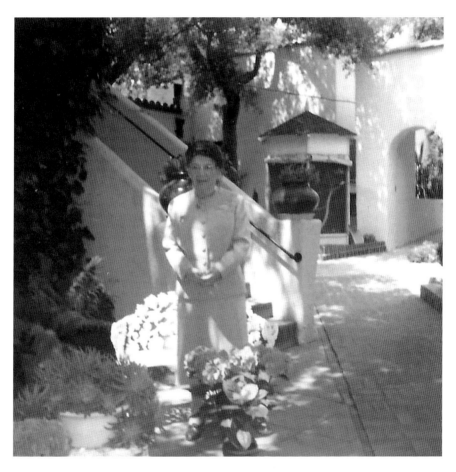

Agnes at Rockhaven in the 1960s. Although she began to slow down during the last years of her life and began handing over more responsibility to her granddaughter, she still remained active in running the property until shortly before her passing in 1967.

Agnes remained a strong but kindhearted leader, but by the late 1950s, she was slowing down. She knew she couldn't run her business forever and entrusted its future to her granddaughter Patricia Traviss, whom she began mentoring. Patricia's assistance couldn't have come at a better time. Agnes was still feisty, but her energy wasn't what it once was, and her blood pressure was now on the high side. It's possible the increasing fatigue was partially to blame for what could have potentially been an embarrassing issue. In 1959, Agnes was indicted on charges of tax evasion for the years 1952, 1953 and 1954. She was accused by Assistant U.S. attorney Robert D. Hornbaker of secretly maintaining a second set of ledgers of business earnings for the purpose of hiding money from the government. Agnes may have been getting older and tired, but she wasn't about to let that accusation stand.

Agnes steadfastly maintained that a clerical error was to blame for the problem, not intentional tax evasion. Her tax returns, she said, were calculated by an outside bookkeeper, and she had followed his instructions on what to pay. When she learned of the discrepancy, she paid $143,485, which included $41,112 in penalties. Judge Ben Harrison ordered Agnes to pay a $9,000 fine, and that closed the matter.

As the 1960s dawned, Patricia's involvement freed Agnes to stay involved in the clubs and charities she liked to work with. Ivan Cole was hired as a horticulturist in 1963 and further enhanced the already lush gardens on the property. His involvement on the grounds would lead to an award-winning landscape. Agnes was still very much involved in Rockhaven's operations, but she wanted to rest more and travel when able, a well-deserved reward for decades of working nonstop.

As she eased herself into semi-retirement, she had one last battle to fight on Rockhaven's behalf. In 1964, the city declared eminent domain to widen Honolulu Avenue, on which Rockhaven had sat for forty-one years. The move not only shaved footage off the property but also ruined the entire front of Rockhaven. The beautiful iron gate that served as an entrance and the decorative rock wall running along the front were removed. It was unattractive and destroyed an entryway specifically designed to positively greet people. A welcoming look and feel were imperative to Rockhaven.

Agnes filed a lawsuit against the city and sued for damages. In addition to the ruined gate and fence, there were monetary issues for rebuilding the property's entrance and property footage lost. City attorney general Henry McClernan recommended settling the suit for $19,000 to pay for the land

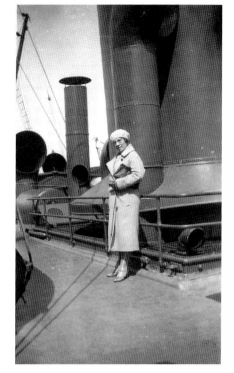

Right: As Agnes began handing over more business responsibilities to her granddaughter, she was finally able to take vacations and travel. Here she is seen on her way to Alaska.

Below: No detail was overlooked when designing Rockhaven's property, including the gate that welcomed residents and visitors. As with the rest of the campus, Agnes insisted that the front gate and surroundings be functional but also beautiful.

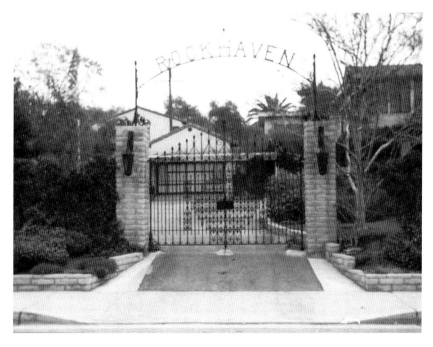

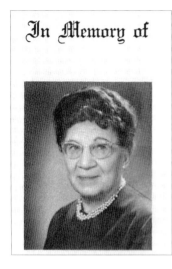

In Memory of

Left: When Agnes passed away in 1967, she was regarded as a pioneer in her community.

Below: In 1964, the city widened Honolulu Avenue, which shaved off square footage from Rockhaven's property and destroyed the front fence and gate. Agnes was furious. Not only had she lost some land, but the beautiful entrance was gone and a chain-link fence left in its place. She sued the city for damages and won $19,000 as compensation for the lost land value and to rebuild the fence.

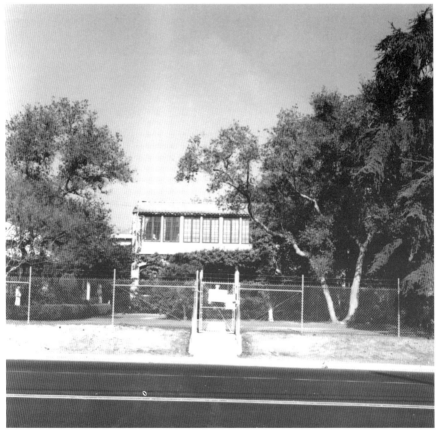

and to repair the gate, wall and landscaping. A new wall and gate were indeed built to once again make visitors and residents feel welcome and safe when entering the property.

Rockhaven's property was once again protected and cared for by its founder. Patricia started taking more ownership and running the daily operations, but Agnes continued to be involved, despite her travels, charity work and age. She only completely stopped her involvement at Rockhaven in July 1967, just one month before passing away of natural causes in August. She was eighty-four years old and a force of nature until the very end. Throughout her life, she had moved to a new country and learned another language. She was a young widow with a baby to support. She worked in asylums. She served the United States in World War I. She went to school and earned a degree. She started her own business and gave back to the community that helped her become a success. She fought for her rights when she needed to. The obituary that ran in the local newspaper called her "a well-known, beloved foothills pioneer," an apt description summing up her life and the way she lived. With all that, she is best remembered for keeping her word and never straying from her promise to provide a safe place where women living with illnesses could recover with respect and dignity.

Chapter 3
Life at Rockhaven

When Agnes Richards moved to Southern California, she had already established a career as a nurse in mental healthcare. She continued on in the same line of work and found conditions similar in California to what she had seen in previous jobs. Although conditions had vastly improved since their inception centuries ago, in the late 1800s and early 1900s, there was still a need for sweeping change.

Life in many sanitariums was hardly the healing medical environment needed for patients seeking recovery in hospitals. Although medical breakthroughs were decades in the future, there were many sanitarium doctors, nurses and staff who still treated their wards inhumanely. It wasn't uncommon to hear stories of abuse, malnourishment, hazardous and substandard conditions, forced physical labor and, in some cases, torture. Some hospitals called their patients "inmates," as though they were in prison.

All patients were vulnerable given their health conditions, but women were especially at risk for predatory male employees or other inmates. Sexual abuse, manipulation and rape were all factors given the poor and unsafe conditions. By today's standards, the word *barbaric* when describing the state of sanitariums before reforms would not be unheard of. It was also fairly easy to have both men and women committed against their will. Cases ranged from the expected, such as manic depression (now called bipolar disorder) and schizophrenia to promiscuity, masturbation, postpartum depression, menopause and, for some especially headstrong women, "noncompliance."

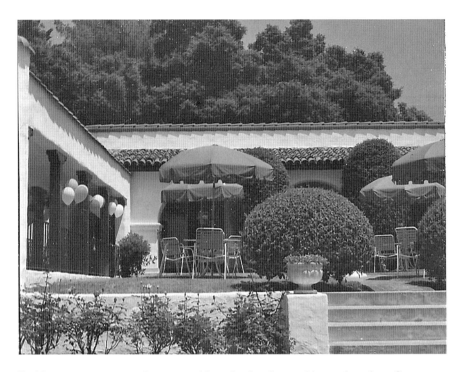

Residents were encouraged to get outside and enjoy the sunshine and gardens. Contact with visiting family members was also considered important for residents to remain mentally healthy. Here, the grounds are decorated for one of the frequent parties for residents and visitors.

None of these factors was lost on Agnes Richards. After observing such conditions firsthand, she was determined that she could run a better facility. During her nursing career, she saw not only what she believed was wrong but also what some facilities did right. This insight enabled her to determine what would work best to help people heal. Furthermore, by founding a hospital that was privately funded, she would be free to form her own rules and care standards.

She began forming her plans in the early 1920s, and by January 1923, her facility was ready to open. Agnes had rented a stone façade house on Honolulu Avenue in the Verdugo hills. Both the location and the house were chosen for distinct reasons. This area of Verdugo City (now Montrose) was already home to other sanitariums. The warm, dry climate, rolling hills and distance from Los Angeles made for an ideal spot. It was far enough away from the big city to provide a peaceful, quiet area and close enough for family to visit and to attract clients.

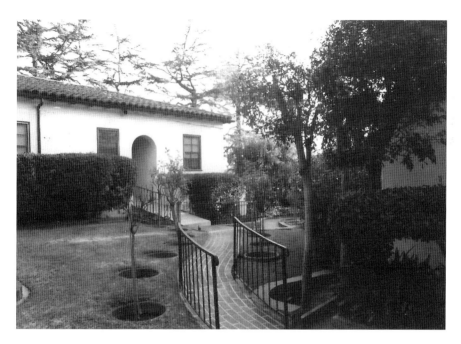

Rockhaven was primarily made up of small houses and bungalows so the residents would feel like they were living in a cozy neighborhood. There were gardens and pathways that meandered around the property. The layout was a direct response to the impersonal, prison-like hospitals that made up most of the mental healthcare hospitals in the United States at the time.

The stone house was also chosen with a distinct purpose in mind. Agnes believed that the mental hospitals she had previously worked in looked foreboding. Instead of giving patients a sense of tranquility, these looming, impersonal structures were intimidating. In contrast, this two-story house had a large, welcoming porch and a balcony. It was surrounded by trellises, mature trees (some were hundreds of years old), pathways and flower beds. Setting women up in an actual house would make them feel like they were *home* and safe. And that's how Agnes chose the name for her new sanitarium: Rockhaven, named for the original rock house she started with and for the safe feeling she was trying to create.

There was one more important element to Rockhaven that Agnes instated from the very beginning: no men. This was a direct response to the cases of sexual abuse that Agnes had learned of earlier in her career. Although doctors in the 1920s were men and there would later be a trusted male gardener, Rockhaven was a place dominated by female employees. It would

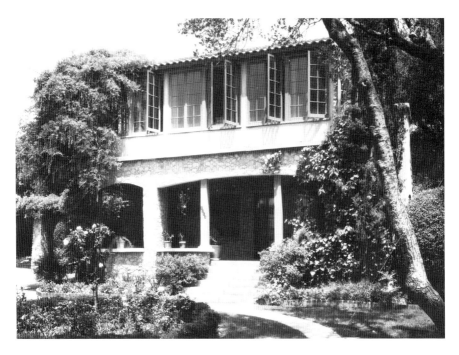

Agnes Richards wanted residents to feel safe while recuperating from their illnesses. One way to accomplish this was to set up her sanitarium in a house. She also permitted only women to enter Rockhaven for treatment. The majority of employees were also women to prevent predatory behavior on vulnerable patients.

be a place where women could live without risk of abuse. Residents, Agnes determined, would all be female.

This provided a sense of peace for mentally and sometimes physically vulnerable women. It also provided a variety of jobs for women, who were limited in career opportunities at the time. As Agnes's sanitarium expanded over the years, more local women found themselves with careers. When Rockhaven opened its doors for business with six female patients in 1923, no one could have predicted that Agnes Richards had just established a business that would be so groundbreaking and ahead its time. She was about to make healthcare and socioeconomic history. Agnes Richards hadn't just opened any ordinary business; she had opened a progressive medical facility that would change mental health for the better, and she was running a business by women, for women, just three years after women won the right to vote and decades before the women's movement.

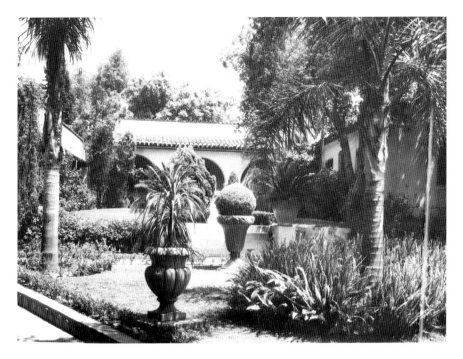

The lush gardens, bungalows and paths ensured that Rockhaven created a peaceful environment for residents. It was designed to distinguish itself from other sanitariums.

Rockhaven was immediately successful, with word spreading that a new private sanitarium catering to women had opened in Verdugo. It wasn't long before Agnes was able to purchase the original stone house and some of the surrounding land. As demand for Rockhaven's services grew, so, too, did the need for more housing. Because Agnes was insistent that Rockhaven feel more like a home than a hospital, she bought a couple of existing bungalows in the area and had them moved to the Rockhaven property. Women shared the small houses, but they had the luxury of just a few women to an actual home. They could step out their front doors and into the sunshine and gardens instead of a hospital hallway.

As business started to boom in the 1930s, it was decided to actually construct, as opposed to buy and then move, buildings to house more residents. The new structures were larger than the little bungalows and more like dormitories, but they still adhered to the homelike setting that Agnes was so determined to achieve. These buildings still had bedrooms, living rooms and small gardens around the houses. A stone fence was built around the

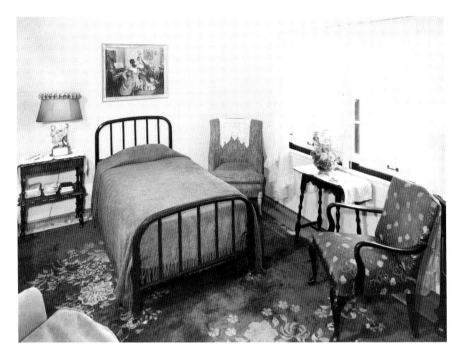

Accommodations for residents were set up as close to a regular home as possible. Bedrooms typically had a similar layout to what one might find in any house.

property, but Agnes took great pride in ensuring that it was beautiful and blended in seamlessly with the surroundings.

Other buildings were also constructed on the premises to accommodate Rockhaven's growth, including a "hospital" structure for women who needed twenty-four-hour care, maintenance buildings, a garage, a professional kitchen and a large dining hall, which was decorated to look like a family dining room. In total, Rockhaven grew to fifteen buildings, and wherever Agnes could incorporate the feeling of a home, she did.

Agnes further took steps to ensure a comfortable environment. No detail was too small, such as referring to the patients as residents or ladies. Although it appeared to be an insignificant gesture, it was a huge step in restoring dignity to the women at Rockhaven. During her time at other sanitariums, Agnes had noticed it was important to keep the human brain active. When patients at standard hospitals were ignored or went untreated, their illnesses got worse. If people were kept physically and mentally active, however, their conditions improved, often significantly. Most of the women

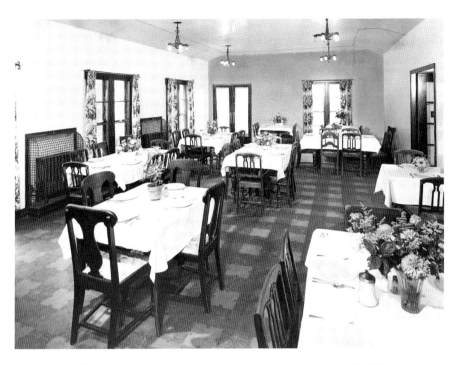

Residents ate dinner together in the dining room, which was designed to feel like a house.

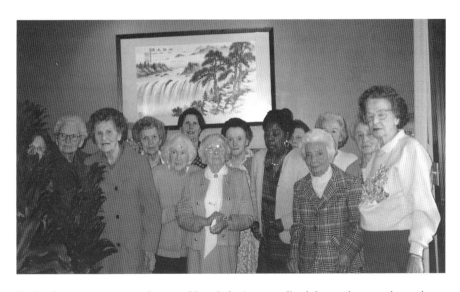

During her years as a nurse in mental hospitals, Agnes realized that patients staying active was imperative when it came to keeping them from retreating into their illnesses. When possible, residents went on outings, such as lunch. The ladies here are out for a Chinese New Year celebration at a local restaurant.

at Rockhaven had mild to moderate "nervous disorders," which ranged from depression and anxiety to mental instability and what was then called nervous breakdowns. Rockhaven also took in women with dementia and more serious mental illnesses, such as schizophrenia. Everyone was treated for the individual ailments, but all were given the same respect and access to the sanitarium's programs.

To keep the ladies active and healthy, Rockhaven arranged for a variety of things to keep them busy. Over Rockhaven's history, the residents gardened, participated in art projects, went out to lunch and had their nails done. The items ladies made were often sold at bazaars to raise addition funds for future projects. In addition to regular visiting hours, there was also a Sunday night "family dinner," to which residents' families were invited. Family participation, in fact, was encouraged. Rockhaven organized parties during the year, often with themes like tropical luaus, with families welcome to attend. Holidays were always celebrated as well. There were Christmas trees during the holidays, Easter parties and lunches out for Valentine's Day, and because most of the women at Rockhaven were mothers, a Mother's Day Tea became a popular annual event. Live entertainment was also sometimes hired as a special treat. Children's groups occasionally visited and sang for the ladies.

Thanks to the efforts of Agnes and the entire staff, residents thrived, and Rockhaven developed a reputation for the highest standard of mental healthcare for women. According to Crescenta Valley historian Mike Lawler, the 1930 census report indicates that forty-four women ranging in age from their twenties up to eighties lived at Rockhaven. Twenty years later in 1950,

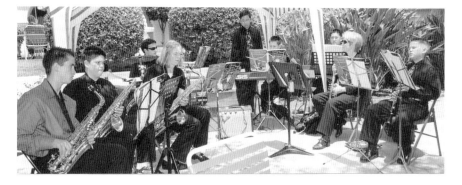

A youth band plays for the residents. Concerts, recitals and entertainment were common for the ladies. Music was especially popular, as Agnes Richards and her granddaughter Patricia Traviss both believed in its healing properties.

the census recorded that number had risen to one hundred women. Business was booming, and families from all walks of life entrusted their loved ones to the women's-only sanitarium. It became known as one of the best facilities money could buy, although Agnes—and later her granddaughter Patricia—tried to keep prices reasonable.

The women at Rockhaven lived there due to a wide variety of issues and ailments. That began to change in the 1960s, which marked the beginning of the radical improvement in mental health medications and treatment. With the advent of antidepressants and anti-anxiety medication, many women were now able to live at home while receiving treatment or recovering from specific bouts of depression and anxiety. Talk therapy also significantly improved since Rockhaven's early days, and it became easier for people to seek out private therapists. Although Rockhaven's population never exclusively became devoted to dementia and what is now recognized as Alzheimer's disease, the women afflicted with these conditions became the majority as time passed.

There were other changes at Rockhaven in the 1960s. As Agnes aged, she began handing off more of the daily responsibilities to her granddaughter Patricia Traviss, though she remained involved to an extent. In fact, Agnes was part of what turned out to be a major turning point in Rockhaven's history when Ivan Cole was hired in 1963 to maintain the gardens. Ivan was a gentle giant originally from Wales and one of the few men employed by Rockhaven. His expertise for gardening and grounds maintenance transformed an already beautiful property to an award-winning landscape.

Thanks to Ivan, Rockhaven won a Los Angeles Beautiful Community Award. Ivan and Agnes both accepted the award at a ceremony that took place at the Statler Hilton Hotel on October 13, 1966. The *Glendale News-Press* wrote about Rockhaven's win the following day on October 14:

> *Exterior landscaping was again praised at Rock Haven* [sic] *Sanitarium. The use of bougainvillea, shrubbery and blossoming trees was described as "particularly enhancing to the neighborhood." Also noted was the statuary arising from a circular rose bed in front of the office. L.A. Beautiful officials said judges look for effective use of water, trees and landscaping when making decisions, coupled with the recognition of what effect a particular building has on its own neighborhood.*

The award was placed proudly in Rockhaven's office. Just a few years later, Rockhaven also won the Glendale Beautiful Award under Ivan, who turned

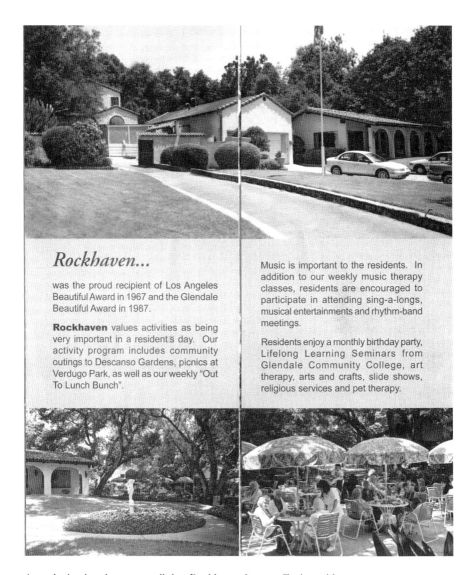

Rockhaven...

was the proud recipient of Los Angeles Beautiful Award in 1967 and the Glendale Beautiful Award in 1987.

Rockhaven values activities as being very important in a resident's day. Our activity program includes community outings to Descanso Gardens, picnics at Verdugo Park, as well as our weekly "Out To Lunch Bunch".

Music is important to the residents. In addition to our weekly music therapy classes, residents are encouraged to participate in attending sing-a-longs, musical entertainments and rhythm-band meetings.

Residents enjoy a monthly birthday party, Lifelong Learning Seminars from Glendale Community College, art therapy, arts and crafts, slide shows, religious services and pet therapy.

A marketing brochure touts all that Rockhaven has to offer its residents.

the gardens of Rockhaven into one of the property's trademark features. He dutifully maintained the grounds (and attended Rockhaven's bazaars and family parties) until he retired in 1997 after thirty-four years of service. But his loyalty to Rockhaven didn't end with his retirement. Rockhaven was sold five years after he retired, and when the property was threatened with demolition in 2007, Ivan Cole, then in his late eighties, spoke to historical

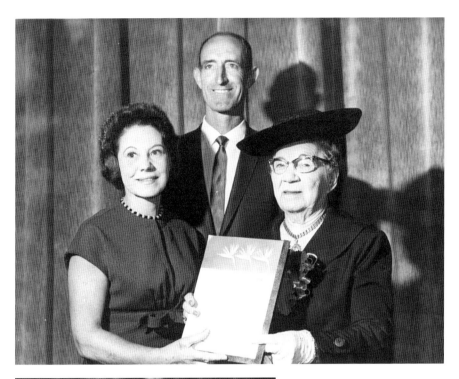

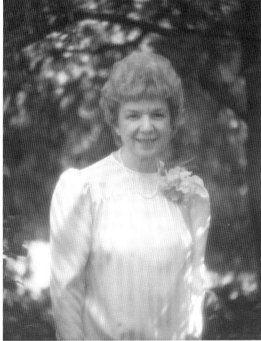

Above: In 1966, Agnes and Rockhaven gardener Ivan Cole accepted the Los Angeles Beautiful Community Award for the property's landscaping. The award hung proudly on a wall in the administration building. Cole was one of the few male employees during Rockhaven's existence. He stayed on as the gardener for nearly three decades.

Left: As the granddaughter of Agnes Richards, Patricia Traviss grew up around Rockhaven. Agnes began mentoring Pat in running the family business during the 1950s. By the 1960s, Pat's responsibilities had increased as her grandmother aged. She finally took over in 1967 and ran the property until she retired in 2001.

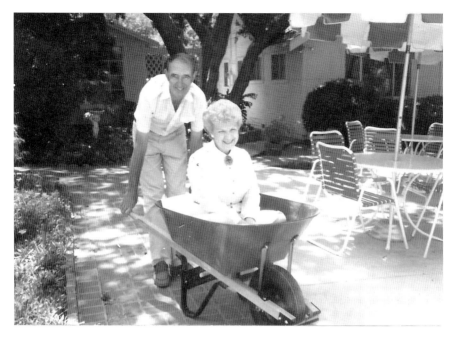

Ivan Cole playfully pushes Patricia Traviss in a wheelbarrow on the Rockhaven grounds.

society members and officials about Rockhaven's local significance. He spoke fondly of Agnes Richards, how well the residents were treated and, of course, the gardens. "I took great pride and was very committed in maintaining the grounds," he told the audience.

Rockhaven was not without its problems, however. In addition to the street widening that destroyed the fence and gobbled up some of the property, the Sylmar earthquake in 1971 significantly damaged the original stone house where Rockhaven started. Agnes had passed away a few years earlier in 1967 and didn't have to bear witness to the sight of the structure's demolition. Patricia, however, was left with no choice but to tear down the now-historic structure. Damages to the old building were beyond repair. In its place was a Spanish-style building with arches that defined a new porch and entrance area. Like her grandmother before her, Patricia's choice in architecture when adding to Rockhaven had a purpose. The buildings on Rockhaven's property dating from the 1930s were constructed in the Spanish style that was popular in Los Angeles at the time. Patricia specifically wanted the architecture to blend together. The new one-story Spanish structure sitting on the original stone house's

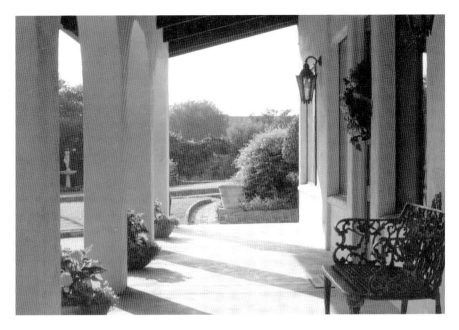

After the original house was torn down, a new administration building was erected in its place. It was constructed in a Spanish style of architecture to match other structures on the property. It retained, however, a welcoming feel, with a porch similar to a house.

spot became the administration building. It remained the administration building until Rockhaven closed for good in 2006.

From 1923 until 2006, thousands of women were treated at Rockhaven with dignity. Families were grateful for the devotion shown to the women who lived there. Employees, including Ivan Cole, staff and nurses, remained loyal and had fond memories. A brochure for Rockhaven once touted, "The tranquil beauty of the gardens, and the opportunity for quiet seclusion—all help to hasten the patient's early recovery."

Agnes Richards set out to create an environment in which women could heal. She did that, but she also made history in the way she treated mental health patients, the successful business she built as a woman and the opportunities she provided to other women for jobs.

Ivan Cole said it best when he spoke to the group trying to save Rockhaven. "This isn't just a place," he told the crowd. "It's a very special place."

Chapter 4

Billie Burke

Actress Billie Burke was destined for a career in entertainment. Born Mary William Ethelbert Appleton Burke on August 7, 1884, in Washington, D.C., "Billie" was the daughter of an ambitious mother, Blanche, who was serious about elevating herself out of the working class. As a widow with four children, Blanche met and married a singer and Barnum & Bailey clown, Billy Burke, at the circus for which he worked in 1883. Their union produced Billie, who, unlike her mother, blossomed into a great beauty as she grew into adulthood. Blanche was well aware that her daughter's pretty face was just one element that could work to her advantage in adulthood.

During childhood, Billie toured the United States and London because of her father's work. While living in London as a youth, Billie was exposed to great elements of culture and, at various times, lived with European families, further exposing her to a higher level of society than her own family's social standing. Meanwhile, Blanche set about arranging for Billie to appear in small roles on the stage.

As Billie studied her craft in London, she remained uninspired by theater life and insisted that she had no desire to become an actress. Mother Blanche had different ideas. In an interview, Blanche was forthcoming about pushing her daughter into acting. "When she says, 'I can't, I can't,' I say, 'Very well, then, if you think you can't, let some other girl have the chance. There are plenty of other girls who would give anything to have the chance you have.'"

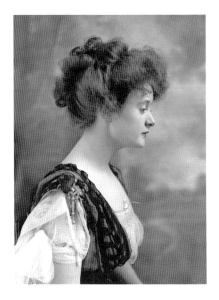

Actress Billie Burke was groomed for life on the stage from an early age. She was considered a delicate beauty in her youth, but her appearance belied a tough personality. Throughout her life, Billie endured a challenging marriage, financial hardship and career changes. She remained the consummate professional despite all the turbulence. *Author's collection.*

As a teen, Billie proved she had talent on the British stage, and her star began to rise in the theater world. Her reputation grew and her career progressed as she performed in London, Paris and New York during the Gilded Age. Critics and audiences alike considered her gifted on the stage and a delicate beauty. It's true that Billie possessed both talent and beauty, but the delicate part applied to her physical features only. She was tougher than she appeared. Then as now, the theater world was a challenging business. Auditioning for parts, getting rejected for jobs, enduring long rehearsals, memorizing dialogue and experiencing the competition among actors created an atmosphere that few people could endure. The skills Billie learned to survive theater life served her just as well in her personal life as they did for work. Like her father, she had a gift for entertaining an audience, but she turned out to be more like Blanche in terms of personality than she probably ever realized. Her ability to persevere and rise above even the most difficult circumstances helped to guide her through an increasingly turbulent life.

As it turns out, her career would be only one aspect of learning to persevere. Life away from the stage proved be just as demanding, if not more so. After meeting and falling deliriously in love with Florenz "Flo" Ziegfeld, the man famous for the follies and theater named in his own honor, Billie realized that life with Flo would be anything but serene. Flo was just as in love with Billie as she was with him, but she learned early in their marriage that he would never be able to overcome his need for attention from women. Over the years, Flo had multiple affairs. His work as the producer of the Ziegfeld Follies guaranteed continual access to entertainment's most beautiful young actresses and dancers. Whether these young women were genuinely charmed by the producer, wanted a job in his popular show or both, Flo ensured that there would never be a shortage of "Ziegfeld Girls" close at hand. Not even the birth of their daughter, Patricia, curbed his enthusiasm for other women.

Hurt as she was by her husband's infidelities, Billie found herself unable to leave her magnetic and—in his own way—very loving husband. Instead of allowing herself to become a victim, Billie relied on her instincts as a fighter. Throughout their entire marriage, Billie remained a devoted wife ready and willing to fend off any serious threats. Young girls could and would come and go, but Billie Burke was the love of Flo Ziegfeld's life, and she knew it—she wasn't going anywhere.

Billie's success on the stage earned her a reputation as a versatile actress. As it turns out, another avenue for work was about to make itself available to accomplished performers of the theater, of which Billie was a premier example. The adaptability she displayed in plays could now be put to use in silent movies, starting in the 1910s. At the time, much of the movie business was still located on the East Coast, so it was an easy commute for New York theater performers. As Billie was a renowned leading lady for theater, it was only natural that movie producers in need of first-rate performers would come calling. Billie acted in silent movies but considered them easy money while in between plays. Movies weren't taken seriously by many, if not most, actors at the time. The general consensus was that movies were a fad, and frankly, they weren't especially challenging for performers who memorized and recited pages of dialogue while also connecting with a live audience. With movies, that in-person connection between performers and crowd disappears.

But producers continued casting Billie when she was available. When movies added sound in 1927, Billie continued to find work in motion pictures. This gives her the rare distinction of making the transition from stage to silent movies to talkies. Many actors and actresses tried and failed to transition from one art form to the other, but that was never the case for Billie Burke. Just as the theater was a different form of acting from silent movies, talkies were also different than the silents in terms of hitting different types of marks and staying close to boom microphones. Each artform required a unique skill set, and Billie managed to master them all. Still, her heart was with the theater, and that's the world where she felt most at home.

Theater life had been good to Billie and Flo, whom she supported when, in February 1927, he opened the opulent Ziegfeld Theater, a building worthy of the large-scale shows bearing the Ziegfeld name. He financed his business venture through tycoon William Randolph Hearst. Although known for his newspaper empire, Hearst was deeply involved in an ongoing affair with actress Marion Davies and, because of her, financed several theater and movie opportunities. As a former Ziegfeld Girl, Davies, and in turn Hearst, would have been familiar with Flo Ziegfeld and his financially successful follies.

The theater was initially a booming success, with landmark runs of *Rio Rita* and *Show Boat*, which ran for 572 performances. But the good fortune for the Ziegfelds did not last. Life for Flo and Billie changed, as it did for most Americans, when the stock market crashed in 1929. It didn't take long for the Great Depression that followed to affect every aspect of the American economy. Elaborate productions and glamorous shows like the ones performed at the Ziegfeld Theater fell out of favor, and Flo could no longer cover his expenses. Suddenly, the once successful Flo was plunged into crippling debt. The burden fell to Billie alone to support the family and try to pay off her husband's creditors. Now she was left with little choice but to leave New York and move permanently to Los Angeles so she could pursue a movie career. The medium once considered a "fad" by so many actors was now proving itself to be the premier entertainment choice for a cash-strapped public. Theater tickets were expensive; movie tickets were priced to accommodate even the smallest budgets. Crowds flocked to movie theaters for relief from the dismal economy.

Once in Los Angeles, Billie had no trouble finding work. She landed roles in sound films as well as in another popular medium, radio. Her first radio role? Performing on a half-hour show called *The Ziegfeld Follies of the Air*.

Billie's life was undergoing one upheaval after another—debt, the theater losing money, leaving stage acting, moving across the country and establishing herself in a new industry. It would have been a challenging adjustment under the best of circumstances, but Billie would have to enter this next phase of her life and career without Flo. He had accompanied her to the West Coast but found himself in ill health and hospitalized at Cedars of Lebanon Hospital in Hollywood. She was working on the set when called to the hospital on behalf of Flo, who died of pleurisy on July 22, 1932. Both Billie and their daughter, Patricia, rushed to the hospital, but neither one of them made it to Flo's side in time. He was dead when they arrived. Billie had believed that her husband's health was improving, so his death came as a shock, and she was devastated by the loss. For all the flaws in their marriage, they had somehow remained devoted to each other. She had built her personal life around Flo, and now suddenly she was alone in what felt like a new world in Los Angeles.

But she had a daughter to think of and Flo's debts to pay. Almost immediately, six lawsuits were filed against Flo's estate. Hearst seized control of the failing Ziegfeld Theater in New York. The Bank of the United States was demanding $37,000 as part of Flo's debt, and there were many other debtors demanding their money. All totaled, Flo's estate owed about $2 million. Drawing on the tough character that had gotten her through so much turmoil in her past, Billie carried on.

Professional luck once again bestowed itself on Billie's career after she was in the Hollywood studio system. Her reputation preceded her, and movies' biggest talents wanted to work with her. "Motion pictures tided me over the most difficult part of my life," she said later. "They were a veritable port in the storm, when my life was going overboard with grief."

She quickly became friends with director George Cukor, who, as the son of an actress, was known for his ability to connect with women and direct his leading ladies to outstanding performances. Cukor eventually cast Billie in her breakout movie role, *Dinner at Eight*, for MGM in 1933. Known for having many of the premier actors and moviemakers under contract, MGM was an ideal place for someone like Billie Burke. She found herself working alongside other theater greats like John and Lionel Barrymore and movie stars of high caliber like Clark Gable, Greta Garbo, Joan Crawford and Jean Harlow.

Dinner at Eight featured an all-star cast and proved itself an excellent vehicle to solidify Billie's reputation in movies. However, George Cukor would later express regret for casting Billie Burke in *Dinner at Eight* as the oblivious character Millicent Jordan. He feared that it had led to her being typecast as a fluttery, airheaded woman when, in actuality, Billie's real personality was nothing of the sort. It's doubtful that *Dinner at Eight* was the primary cause of the types of roles she was offered, but she did indeed fill a certain type of role when needed. Still, a middle-aged Billie was working steadily in Hollywood at a time when most leading ladies were groomed in their teens.

When she was cast in her now-signature role as Glinda the Good Witch in *The Wizard of Oz* (1939), Billie was fifty-four years of age. She looked nowhere near fifty-four; the beauty that had served her so well in her youth continued into middle age. In contrast, character actress Margaret Hamilton, who played the Wicked Witch of the West, was just thirty-six during the filming of the movie and looked older than Billie.

After *The Wizard of Oz*, the movie's success guaranteed Billie a level of career stability that few actresses enjoyed. She continued working in movies into her old age. She needed the work. As late as 1940, eight years after Flo's death, she was forced to liquidate many of her assets. She had to sell off belongings from their mansion in New York and then finally the house itself for significantly less than it was worth because of the loans against it.

In addition to movies, she continued working in radio and even dabbled in theater, although three of the five plays she appeared in after Flo's death revolved around the Ziegfeld Follies theme.

Ziegfeld themes came up in other ways. In 1936, MGM produced a movie about Flo Ziegfeld called, appropriately enough, *The Great Ziegfeld*. William Powell starred as Flo, and some actors even played themselves. One who did not, however, was Billie Burke. Myrna Loy, who had been successfully cast opposite Powell in the Thin Man series of movies, played Billie. Despite being Flo's widow, MGM consulted her very little with fact-checking or research. The studio promised her a portion of the box office earnings, but she had very little to do with the movie itself. When it was completed, she refused to watch it and didn't see it until it ran on television years later. As for Myrna Loy, Billie said, "She doesn't look much like me, does she?"

Billie's career continued on successfully, but now there was one more medium to conquer: television. From the summer of 1951 to the spring of 1952, Billie hosted *At Home with Billie Burke*. Only one episode survives, so little is known about the show, but it gave Billie the distinction of being one of television's first female talk show hosts. For all her accomplishments, however, there was a noticeable change in Billie by the late 1950s. People on the set noticed that she was starting to have difficulty remembering lines. Billie had memorized countless pages of dialogue over her decades-long career, so this was a first. It became such an issue that Billie retired after making a movie called *Pepe* in 1960. She was now in her mid-seventies and had worked almost nonstop for the majority of her life. She had successfully paid back her husband's debts and conquered theater, movies, radio and television.

It was reported that Billie was showing signs of dementia, but she denied this and said she retired because "acting wasn't fun anymore." She lived quietly in Beverly Hills, where she surrounded herself with memories such as pictures and a bust of Flo, the husband she missed so much. She attended church and wrote a memoir.

Eventually, Billie was moved to Rockhaven, where she was treated for dementia. Today, she might be diagnosed with Alzheimer's disease, but during the 1960s, no such diagnosis existed. She passed away on May 14, 1970. Her daughter, Patricia, asked George Cukor, the director who had been such a loyal friend to Billie, to speak at the memorial. She is buried in New York next to her beloved Flo, finally joining him in death as she had been in life. Her modest marker reads "Billie Burke Ziegfeld."

Chapter 5

Gladys Monroe, the Mother of a Hollywood Legend

Marilyn Monroe is one of the world's most recognizable faces, transcending her movie star fame and achieving the rare status of icon. Millions of people can immediately identify the wavy platinum blond hair, the beauty mark on her left check and the bright red lipstick. Many fans are also familiar with at least some of the mythology that has sprung up around Marilyn's Cinderella-like story: born with the name Norma Jeane to a mentally unstable mother, shuffling around from various foster homes to an orphanage, reinventing herself as the glamorous movie star Marilyn Monroe and living on in photos and on screen.

What is less commonly known is her relationship with her mother, Gladys, and her family's history of mental illness. Marilyn herself struggled with anxiety and depression, but one of her greatest fears as an adult was succumbing to mental illness like her mother. Marilyn had cause for concern, as serious mental health issues ran in her family and can be traced back at least as far as Marilyn's great-grandfather Tilford Hogan.

Tilford, born on February 24, 1851, was a midwestern farm laborer who married at least twice, producing four living children. Not a whole lot is known about his life, but his death certificate indicates that he committed suicide by hanging on May 27, 1933, in Missouri at the age of eighty-two. He outlived three of his four children, including his daughter Della Mae (Marilyn's maternal grandmother), who had preceded him in death in 1927.

It was Della Mae's lineage that would produce Gladys Monroe and later the actress Marilyn Monroe. Della, born in Missouri on July 1, 1876, was described as a vivacious and mischievous young girl. Her parents made the unusual decision for the era to divorce when she was thirteen years old, and she bounced between her parents. In 1898, she met a house painter from Indiana named Otis Monroe, who talked of studying painting in Europe. His dreams of studying the great masters would never come to pass, but he was successful in wooing Della. The two married in 1899 and soon began a fairly nomadic existence around the country in search of work.

In 1901, Otis accepted a job working for the Mexican National Railway in Mexico, not far from the Texas border. On May 27, 1902, Della delivered the first of their two children, a daughter named Gladys Pearl Monroe, while living in Mexico. The family's stay across the border did not last long, however, and by the spring of 1903, the Monroes had moved back to the United States when Otis accepted a job with Pacific Electric Railway (also called Red Cars), a private mass transit system that utilized streetcars and buses to connect the expanding population in Southern California, including the counties of Los Angeles, Riverside, San Bernardino and Orange. The family settled in Los Angeles, where a second child, a son named Marion Otis Monroe, was born in 1904.

Life for the family continued in an unstable pattern. Once in Southern California, they moved several times per year, a habit that prevented Gladys and Marion from feeling secure or developing friendships. Furthermore, Otis was known to drink heavily, so when his memory began failing, it was not too much of a surprise, at least initially. But his health continued to deteriorate rapidly, and it became clear that there was a problem much more severe than just drinking. Painful migraines, shakes and violent rages began to frighten Della and the children. As dementia overtook him, Otis was admitted in 1908 to Patton State Hospital, a psychiatric facility in San Bernardino County, where he was diagnosed with syphilis. He died unable to recognize his family at Patton in 1909 at the age of forty-three.

Although there was an explanation for Otis Monroe's death, his wife and children were mistakenly convinced that he had died of hereditary insanity. Life for Della, Gladys and Marion only continued to unravel. Della, believing that Marion should have a man's influence, sent her son to live with relatives in San Diego. She also remarried to one of her deceased husband's co-workers at Pacific Electric, but the union crumbled within two years.

Della and Gladys found themselves at a boardinghouse in Venice Beach within walking distance of the Pacific Ocean. Della was also dating again, this time to a suitor with whom teenage Gladys did not get along. Unlike her average-looking mother, fourteen-year-old Gladys was growing into a beautiful young woman and soon had a suitor of her own in Jasper Baker, a native Kentuckian in his mid-twenties. When Gladys discovered she was pregnant by this older gentleman, Della hatched a solution—marrying her teenage daughter off, which would in turn make her free to pursue her own relationship. Gladys's age was fudged on official paperwork to make her appear older, and she married Jasper (listed as John Baker on the marriage certificate) on May 22, 1917, just five days short of her fifteenth birthday.

Gladys and Jasper's son, Robert Baker, nicknamed Jackie, was born on January 16, 1918. A daughter, Berniece, followed in July 1919. The marriage turned out to be a disaster. Young Gladys was likely not prepared to care for children. Jackie reportedly nearly lost an eye when she placed broken glass in a trash can that was within the toddler's reach.

For his part, Jasper was known to verbally and physically abuse Gladys, including once whipping her across the back with a horse bridle after she spoke too long with one of his brothers. During an argument that turned physical in the front seat of a car between husband and wife, Jackie accidentally opened the door of the backseat and fell out onto the street from the moving vehicle. Deciding she'd had enough, Gladys filed for divorce in 1921, and it was finalized in 1922. Unfortunately for Gladys, it was not the end of her drama with Jasper, who kidnapped their two children and moved with them to his native Flat Lick, Kentucky. Devastated, Gladys traveled to Kentucky in pursuit of her children, even settling in town and working as a housekeeper for a family with young children, including a little girl named Norma Jean.

Jasper remarried, this time to an older and more matronly woman, and the stepmother set about raising Jackie and Berniece. Unable to regain custody of her children, Gladys became disillusioned and reluctantly moved home to Los Angeles, which was now a city rapidly expanding in population. The movies had also come to town, and Gladys found work in the burgeoning industry as a film cutter.

Only in her early twenties and still beautiful, Gladys worked days and spent her nights living the life of a flapper—dancing, drinking and dating. Her co-worker and best friend, Grace McKee, was a frequent cohort in her adventures. They were also movie fans, which seems natural considering their line of work.

Concerned with her daughter's partying lifestyle, Della strongly encouraged Gladys to try settling down. Gladys married for a second time, this time to Martin Edward Mortensen, on October 14, 1924, in Los Angeles. Mortensen, also marrying for the second time, was in his mid-twenties and worked for the gas company. In theory, he was a good match for Gladys, but she apparently wasn't finished sowing her oats and almost immediately grew bored with her husband. Not long after marrying, the couple separated, and Gladys resumed her life of dancing and drinking out on the town with Grace.

Work life also provided the opportunity to find a boyfriend, as Gladys caught the eye of a supervisor at Consolidated Film, where she was employed. Charles Stanley Gifford, who went by Stan, was by all accounts a handsome and charming man. Gladys succumbed to his charms, and the two started dating in 1925. Around Christmas of that same year, Gladys discovered that she was once again expecting a baby.

Stan's response was hardly enthusiastic, and he commented that it was a good thing Gladys was already married, implying that her estranged husband could be listed on the birth certificate to hide the fact that the baby was illegitimate. Stan, who was recently divorced and had a young son with his ex-wife, wanted no part of having to serve as father to yet another kid. Soon after receiving Gladys's news, Stan Gifford quit his Hollywood job and moved out to the small community of Hemet to open a dairy. He never returned, leaving a pregnant Gladys alone.

When Gladys gave birth on June 1, 1926, she delivered her daughter, named Norma Jeane, in the charity ward of Los Angeles General Hospital. Gladys took Stan's suggestion and named her estranged husband as the baby's father on the birth certificate to avoid stigma. Less than two weeks later, Gladys placed Norma Jeane with neighbors of her mother, Della, in the Los Angeles suburb of Hawthorne. Gladys felt she couldn't properly care for her infant as a single parent, and Wayne and Ida Bolender were known for taking in foster children.

Wayne and Ida soon took in another baby, a boy named Lester, who was born in August, just two months after Norma Jeane. Because Norma Jeane and Lester were so close in age, the Bolenders not only raised them as siblings but even called them "the twins." Gladys visited on occasion and sometimes took Norma Jeane on outings, but life with the Bolenders was a stark contrast to how Gladys lived. The Bolenders were deeply religious and eschewed activities like dancing, card playing, movies, smoking and drinking. Outward appearances were modest, especially for women, who were expected to keep jewelry to a minimum, not wear cosmetics and wear their hair up. Gladys, on the other hand, not only loved all these things, but some of her day visits with Norma Jeane included trips to the movies and appointments at a salon.

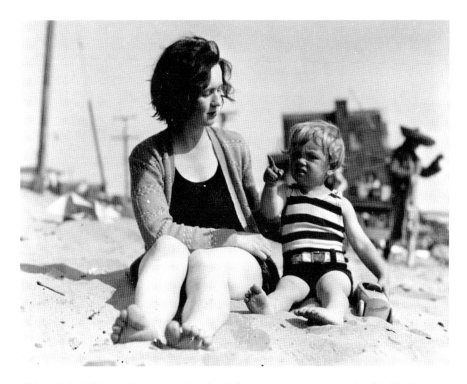

Although little Norma Jeane was placed with foster parents at two weeks old, Gladys visited with her daughter when possible. Day trips included the movies, beauty parlors and lunch. On this particular day, mother and daughter are enjoying a day at Venice Beach. *Author's collection.*

Still, the Bolenders provided a stable environment for Norma Jeane, who sang in a children's choir for a sunrise Easter service at the Hollywood Bowl one year. But despite the home Wayne and Ida provided for her, the Monroe family was still a part of her life. Gladys visited, and Della lived across the street. (As an adult, Marilyn Monroe recalled that her grandmother tried to smother her with a pillow while in her crib. The only verification of this story is from Marilyn herself. If true, it would mean that she had to have been an infant at the time and therefore was *told* about the incident when she got older, because she would have been too young to remember the smothering.)

What can be verified, however, is that Della did break into the Bolenders' house when Norma Jeane was ten months of age. In a documentary filmed in 1964, Wayne and Ida were interviewed about their former foster daughter. Ida recalled, "[Della] did come over one

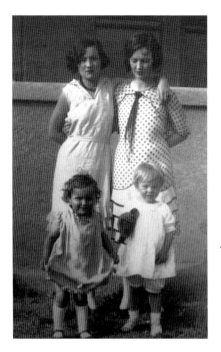

A picture of the Monroe family in 1928. On the left, Olive Monroe stands behind her toddler, Ida Mae Monroe. Gladys Monroe Baker, *right*, stands behind her toddler, Norma Jeane. Olive was married to Marion Monroe, the younger brother of Gladys Monroe. In 1929, Marion left for work one day and never returned, leaving Olive and their three young children alone and destitute. It was believed that Marion was suffering from schizophrenia, a diagnosis his sister Gladys would one day share. *Author's collection.*

day for no reason that I know of and broke in the glass on our front door. And I believe we called the police."

Just a couple of months later, Della Mae Monroe died at Norwalk State Hospital on August 23, 1927. Her cause of death was myocarditis (heart disease), with "manic depressive psychosis" also listed as a contributing factor.

That was not the end of the mental health story for the Monroe family. Della's son (and Gladys's brother) Marion Monroe left for work one day in 1929 and never returned. Marion, by then married and the father of three small children (ages four, two and seven months), abandoned his family, which left them destitute. Although his wife, Olive, filed a claim with the missing persons bureau and her mother hired a private detective, Marion was never seen or heard from again. Olive was forced to begin legal proceedings to declare Marion dead and petition the county of Los Angeles for welfare, which was the only option available for her in that era. It is now generally believed that Marion likely suffered from paranoid schizophrenia, which probably spurred him to disappear.

Things for the family were about to take another turn when Wayne and Ida Bolender requested to adopt Norma Jeane when she was about seven years old. They had adopted Lester and also wanted to formally make his "twin," Norma Jeane, an official part of their family. Perhaps fearing the loss of another child, Gladys refused to sign adoption papers and used this moment as a reason to regain custody of her daughter. Gladys removed Norma Jeane from the only home she had known and from her "brother."

Determined to set up a proper home for herself and Norma Jeane, Gladys decided to buy a house. Her best friend, Grace, strongly advised against taking on a commitment as big as a mortgage while getting reacquainted with her daughter. Gladys ignored this good advice and purchased a three-bedroom house near the Hollywood Bowl. She still dreamed of regaining custody of her other two children, and she wanted enough room for all of them. She also wanted all three of her children to have the same last name—Baker—so Gladys changed Norma Jeane's surname from Mortenson to Baker.

Gladys's dreams of family life, however, would never come true. She struggled to pay the mortgage and had to rent out part of the house to boarders, an English couple who worked as actors. She also found herself in the role of mother, which in and of itself was new for her. Not only that, but she had to work and raise the child by herself.

The strain on Gladys worsened considerably in 1933, when she learned of the back-to-back deaths of her grandfather by suicide in May and of her estranged fifteen-year-old son, Jackie, of tuberculosis of the kidneys in August. Gladys's emotional health crumbled rapidly. She was severely depressed and had difficulty expressing affection for anyone, including for her daughter. In retrospect, she was showing signs of the mental illness that would plague her for the rest of her life.

In January 1935, Gladys suffered a complete mental breakdown. The English couple tried in vain to help and calm her down. With no alternative, the boarders were forced to call an ambulance and watch as Gladys was forcibly escorted from her home. Norma Jeane returned home from school that day to find her mother gone, never to return. Her mother was very sick, she was told, and she wouldn't be able to see her for a long time. It was a trauma the eight-year-old girl seemed to have trouble recovering from. Mother and daughter's time together was brief, and a maternal bond never had time to develop. It never would.

Gladys was admitted to Norwalk State Hospital, the very same psychiatric hospital where her mother had died a few years earlier in a manic-depressive psychosis. Doctors at Norwalk diagnosed Gladys with paranoid schizophrenia, an illness that expresses itself differently in each person, though there are some common symptoms. Gladys displayed several, including a preoccupation with religion (in her case, Christian Science) and delusions (for her it was persecution).

On January 15, 1935, Gladys was "adjudged insane." Ever the loyal friend, Grace began legal proceedings to become Norma Jeane's permanent guardian. It was Grace who arranged foster care for Norma Jeane. When Norma Jeane wasn't living with Grace herself, Grace placed her with trusted friends and family. Grace also assumed the unenviable task of cataloging all of Gladys's possessions so she could sell them off and pay her friend's debts.

Gladys spent the rest of her life in and out of sanitariums and rest homes, but her illness ensured life was never peaceful for her. On January 20, 1937, Gladys escaped from a guard's custody in Altascadero, California, during a transfer from Norwalk State Hospital to Portland, Oregon. When she finally made contact with her oldest surviving child, Berniece, her letters were so rambling and confusing that the now-adult daughter wondered if her long-lost mother had brain damage.

At points in the 1940s, Gladys did try to live outside the walls of psychiatric hospitals, with varying degrees of success. One such time included the summer of 1946, when she moved into a duplex with Grace's aunt Ana Lower, along with Norma Jeane (now modeling and trying to break into movies) and Berniece, who, along with her young daughter Mona Rae, was attempting to get to know her mother and half sister with an extended visit in Los Angeles.

At the end of the summer, Berniece returned home to her husband and Gladys went to Oregon, only to return to Los Angeles a few months later. She married for the last time in 1949 to John Eley, who, it turns out, was still technically married to his previous wife. He and Gladys still lived in Los Angeles as man and wife until he died in 1952. She bounced around in institutions until 1953, when Grace suggested to the now-successful actress Marilyn Monroe (who was using her mother's maiden name as her own) that she place her mother into a private facility that could better care for Gladys's needs.

At Grace's suggestion, Marilyn placed her mother in Rockhaven Sanitarium in February 1953. It was likely one of the last acts of friendship on Grace's part, as she died from a barbiturate overdose on September 28 of that year. Grace had a heart condition and suffered from alcoholism and pill addiction. It is unclear if Marilyn knew the circumstances surrounding Grace's death because at the time, it was believed that Grace had cancer. Berniece later recalled that she thought Grace's death was cancer-related and it wasn't until 1979 that she discovered the truth. Having requested to see Grace's death certificate, Berniece was shocked to see that the manner of death was suicide.

Marilyn paid for her mother's monthly care at Rockhaven, even going so far as to set up a trust. It is unknown if Marilyn actually visited Gladys at Rockhaven, but it seems unlikely, given they had never bonded as mother and daughter. Although Marilyn assumed responsibility for her mother, she never felt especially close to her. Most likely, Marilyn sent her business manager, Inez Melson, to visit with Gladys at Rockhaven.

At Rockhaven, Gladys enjoyed the amenities to which other residents also had access. She participated in crafts, knitted and studied the Bible. In November 1959, with Marilyn's consent, Inez filed a petition with the court to be named as Gladys Eley's conservator. A few weeks later in December, Los Angeles Superior Court judge Burdette Daniels granted the request and named Inez Melson as Gladys's legal guardian. At the time, Marilyn was married to playwright Arthur Miller and living on the East Coast, so she was not present for any of the proceedings.

When Marilyn died on August 5, 1962, the now-divorced movie star was once again living in Los Angeles. Gladys was not told immediately of her youngest child's death, but it is clear that at some point Gladys was informed and even comprehended the loss. In a letter to Inez postmarked August 22, 1962, Gladys wrote, "I am very grateful for your kind and gracious help toward Berniece and myself and to dear Norma Jeane. She is at peace and at rest now and may Our God bless her & help her always. I wish you to know that I gave her [Norma] Christian Science treatments for approximately one year."

After Marilyn's death, it was determined that Gladys would stay at Rockhaven. Although she was receiving high-quality care, Gladys's mental health still made her stay at Rockhaven difficult at times. On July 4, 1963, Gladys knotted a bedsheet and dropped it out her window so she could climb out and escape to freedom. It was a first-floor window, and she could have just as easily walked out her own door. Nevertheless, the escape plan worked—at least temporarily. She was found about twenty-four hours later hiding in the boiler room of Lakeview Baptist Terrace Church, located ten miles away from the sanitarium. In her hands were a Bible and a Christian Science handbook.

She must have walked there, and authorities determined she had probably spent the night in the church. When the media learned of the story, photographers snapped Gladys's picture and splashed photos of Marilyn

Monroe's mentally ill mother all over the newspapers. J. Brian Reid, who was pastor of the church Gladys had been found hiding in, was considerably kinder to the mentally ill woman than the media. When reporters asked him for a quote, he replied, "She was very calm and cool, the kind of person to whom your heart goes out."

It's unknown why Gladys tried to escape, whether it was a response of grief after her daughter's passing or if it was simply a pattern, as she had tried to escape before. What is clear is that Gladys's bill at Rockhaven was overdue and unpaid.

Marilyn's will was signed and dated January 14, 1961, with an estate valued at $1 million. After Marilyn's death, her will revealed that she had left her mother a trust of $100,000 with $5,000 to be paid per year for Gladys's care. This was an extension of the trust that Marilyn had set up during her lifetime in order to pay for Gladys's stay at Rockhaven. Despite the increasing value in Marilyn's estate due to television interest in her movies, her will wasn't able to pay out for a number of years due to heavy taxes and creditors. (Paula Strasberg, for example, was owed $22,200 for acting coach services, and Joe DiMaggio was owed $5,000 for a loan that was used as a down payment for Marilyn's house in Los Angeles. Her agents also filed the largest claim for $80,168.) The lack of funds also meant there was no money with which to pay Gladys's bill, which in theory meant that she could have been asked to leave. The staff at Rockhaven permitted her to stay for free for the time being.

By July 1965, Marilyn Monroe's estate owed Rockhaven $4,133 in back payments for Gladys's $425-per-month bill. Around this time, Rockhaven received an envelope with a handwritten message that read, "Put this on Marilyn's mother's bill." Inside were two $1 bills. The note was likely from Inez Melson, who was executrix of Marilyn's estate, and was quoted in a newspaper article as saying that was all the estate had received so far and that "the sanitarium, which has been so nice, isn't going to set her out on the street."

Inez Melson and Marilyn's attorneys, Aaron Frosch (executor of the estate) and Milton Rudin, continued working with Rockhaven through the mid-1960s. Reporter Earl Wilson wrote in his syndicated newspaper column dated June 21, 1965, that "although Marilyn, in death, still earns about $150,000 a year in deferred salaries, and while her total earnings, including movie sales to TV, have come to over $800,000, virtually all is going for taxes. There have been no business expenses to deduct and Marilyn's continuing income is taxed at the highest bracket, 70 per cent.

There were also back federal income taxes of $118,000 to be paid for 1958 to 1962."

At some point in 1965, Aaron Frosch made two payments on behalf of Marilyn Monroe Productions totaling $2,547 against the outstanding Rockhaven bill. Inez, who visited with Gladys at Rockhaven regularly, further went on record by correcting information about Rockhaven and praising the sanitarium's treatment of her. "There have been reports in some foreign papers that she is being humiliated because she is in a public ward at the hospital, but these are untrue. Mrs. Eley is an ambulatory patient—she walks around. She has always shared a room with another patient. Even very wealthy patients live in rooms for two people. The institution officials have been kind and generous and she is as contented there as one who is ill can be."

Inez further made the point that Gladys did not read newspapers, so it was difficult to say if she knew of the problems with her bill. Certainly, Inez Melson and Aaron Frosch were trying to work with Rockhaven on Gladys's behalf, and the efforts appear to have kept the elderly woman happy and in a safe environment. As Marilyn's taxes and debts were paid off, the income her movies continued to make eventually paid back the money owed to Rockhaven in full. "Marilyn's mother and I go shopping at least once a month," Inez said. "Nobody seeing us having lunch would ever suspect that the little white-haired woman who once looked like Marilyn is actually Marilyn's mother. Her only concern, since she doesn't read the newspapers, is for her religious books."

But Gladys's illness took a dark turn the following year. In April and then again in May 1966, Gladys attempted suicide at Rockhaven by trying to stifle herself with bedsheets. "My soul has gone to God, my body might as well go also," she said.

The matter was larger than just Rockhaven's jurisdiction, and the case ended up in front of a jury, which determined that Gladys was a danger to herself and others. A newspaper article from September 1966 indicated that Gladys would need to move from Rockhaven to a California state mental institution designed for higher-risk patients. It is likely not what Marilyn would have wanted for her mother. Although she was no longer able to step in on Gladys's behalf, another daughter was—Berniece Baker Miracle.

In November 1966, Berniece had Gladys released to her custody instead of a state-run institution. Gladys moved from California to Florida to reside with her daughter's family. As in Los Angeles, where Gladys sometimes lived in facilities and other times in the outside world, Gladys at times stayed with her daughter and son-in-law. She also lived on occasion in a nursing home. Gladys passed away in Gainesville from heart failure on March 11, 1984. Her remains were cremated, and there was a small memorial for family, close friends and Christian Science associates. Her final resting place is unknown to the public, per her request.

Gladys Monroe's life was marked by illness—both her own and her family members'. In the end, what she most wanted was to be a mother to her children, two of whom she outlived. In a roundabout way, Gladys's wish to be reunited with her daughter Berniece came true. It was much later than she anticipated or hoped, but Berniece was there when Gladys needed her the most and cared for her at the end.

Chapter 6

The Women of Clark Gable

During his long career and decades before Elvis Presley swung his hips on the *Ed Sullivan Show*, Clark Gable was known as "the King." When Elvis later became known as the King of Rock 'n' Roll or simply the King, Clark Gable's nickname was refined to the King of Hollywood. Regardless of the updated title, Clark Gable lived up to the King moniker.

As a leading man for decades, Clark Gable had a distinguished career that included an Academy Award for Best Actor in *It Happened One Night* and a career-defining role as Rhett Butler in *Gone with the Wind*. He has the very rare distinction of being one of the few Hollywood icons who is still a recognized and bankable star today, even decades after his death.

Clark Gable's private life was closely tied to women, as he didn't like to be alone. To understand his choices in women and how deeply attached he could become to them, one must look at his childhood. William Clark Gable was born on February 1, 1901, in Cadiz, Ohio, to a modest family. His father, William "Will" Gable, was an oil well driller. His mother, Adeline, died when Clark was just ten months old. Although her official cause of death was listed as an epileptic seizure, it's possible that she had a brain tumor. Will Gable remarried a few years later to a woman named Jennie, who raised little Billy (as he was then known) as her own, but the loss of his biological mother appears to have made a lasting impact on him. He would feel the need to be "mothered" by women or receive attention from them his entire adult life.

Will Gable was a rugged man who insisted his son learn skills like hunting, fishing and manual labor, all of which he continued to pursue as an adult. His stepmother, on the other hand, balanced out his education by teaching Billy how to play the piano and the importance of personal grooming and dressing well. From an early age, Billy excelled at both skill sets. He was a fine hunter and loved working on cars. He also loved playing music, including brass instruments and the piano, and reciting Shakespeare.

After getting a job at Firestone Tire and Rubber Company in Akron, it looked as though Billy might follow in his father's working-class shoes. But secretly, the gawky and shy Billy longed for the stage. Emboldened by an inheritance at the age of twenty-one, Billy Gable was finally free to pursue his dream of acting as a career.

Billy began finding work in small theater companies. It was a life that required travel, and he made his way around the Midwest and finally to Oregon, supporting himself along the way with odd jobs such as logging and necktie sales. The tools that his father and stepmother had instilled were serving him well as he worked toward his bigger career goal.

While living in Portland, Oregon, he met an acting coach named Josephine Dillon. It was under Josephine's tutelage that Billy Gable would change from a shy, awkward-looking boy working in second-rate theater companies into a mass market leading man named Clark Gable.

The Star Maker: Josephine Dillon

Born on January 26, 1884, in Denver, Josephine Dillon's background had very little in common with her future student and husband's humble roots. Her father, Henry Clay Dillon, was a Denver-area judge who later went on to work as a district attorney in Los Angeles. Her mother was a prominent socialite, and her older sister—Josephine was one of six children—was an accomplished opera singer. Before launching into a career in theater and as an acting coach, Josephine herself was educated in Los Angeles and Europe and at Stanford University. She studied acting in Italy and worked on Broadway before turning her career from acting to teaching. She set up her own school in Portland, which is where she met none other than William Clark Gable.

There are various stories about how the two met, but Clark Gable himself said in a 1938 newspaper article that in Portland he worked for the phone company, a job that would lead him directly to his first wife. Josephine's business required service from the telephone company, and Billy Gable happened to be the employee sent out on the job. And he knew exactly who the boss was when he got there. He recalled:

> *Early in the spring of 1924 we picked up a hurry call from the Little Theater. The stage director, Miss Josephine Dillon, reported a wire out of order and I went over to fix it. I had read about her in the newspapers. She had been [a] leading woman for Edward Everett Horton and she had played Broadway.*
>
> *Miss Dillon listened very patiently to my story, while I worked on that disconnected wire. She was one of the kindest persons I had ever met and I must have put up considerable argument as to why I belonged in her stock company. She heard me out and even encouraged me to make another stab at theater.*

From that moment on, Josephine become Billy's teacher and mentor, eventually even serving as a benefactor and, finally, a romantic partner. She was seventeen years older than the eager aspiring actor. Under her direction, Billy began exercises to improve in the craft of acting. Together, they worked on improving his timing and diction. She also guided him through a complete physical transformation. With Josephine's help, he learned how a better diet and exercise would improve his body. With practice, he started to lower his speaking voice. She even paid to fix his teeth, which were in very poor condition.

Years later, after they were divorced, Josephine recalled what she first saw in the raw actor to newspaper columnist Adela Rogers St. John:

> *I saw potential as soon as he walked on the stage in that stock company in Portland, but I think he was—he knew less than any other young actor I ever worked with. Oh, yes. The fire was there. The tremendous desire. I was sure of the strength and stamina for the hard work and self-discipline which makes an actor, and Clark Gable is a fine actor. The only thing that bothered me—I was not sure just at first that he was teachable.*

Josephine Dillon created the foundation for the ultimate male movie star. She also created the foundation for the women Clark Gable would gravitate to for the rest of his life: the boy whose biological mother died when he was too young to form memories of her would forever look for women who were older, more worldly or both. He also liked when women doted on him, and Josephine filled all these needs.

When Billy's physical characteristics and acting abilities had sufficiently improved, the couple decided to head to Hollywood together. The move also meant uprooting Josephine's business. Her reputation was respected enough that when she moved to Los Angeles it warranted a mention in the July 13, 1924 edition of the *Los Angeles Times*, which wrote, "Josephine Dillon, dramatic coach, has come to Los Angeles from New York, and will teach here. Her work consists of oral expression, play directing and preparing students for stage and screen careers. Out of her class she will develop material for a Little Theater Guild, which will present plays of the better sort."

She was actually arriving by way of Portland, where Billy remained for five months. Due to the societal customs of the 1920s, they couldn't move at the same time or live together unless married. After Billy arrived, they were married in Los Angeles on December 16, 1924. He was twenty-three and she was forty, but their marriage certificate incorrectly stated that he was twenty-four and she was thirty-four.

During the next few years, Josephine continued to help Billy—now Clark—with his career and acting lessons. He began picking up jobs in films as an extra or bit parts. Finding work for actors became even more competitive after the stock market crash of 1929, which brought about the Great Depression and, subsequently, the cancelation of several plays. The theater world was now flooded with out-of-work actors. Clark was lucky enough to find work in Los Angeles in the 1930 production of *The Last Mile*. The role brought him enough positive attention that MGM took notice of him and inquired about signing him to a contract. After years of hard work, Clark Gable was officially a rising star in Hollywood.

But there was one problem: Josephine Dillon, the wife who had dedicated herself to building her husband up physically, emotionally and professionally. Despite her talent in creating Clark Gable, who was about to become a motion picture heartthrob, she was significantly older than her now-dashing husband. Worse, she was matronly. A leading man couldn't be seen with an old, plain woman on his arm while attending glamorous movie premieres or making public appearances. He had also become romantically involved with another woman. The awkward Billy Gable had not only transformed himself into the leading man named Clark Gable but had also turned into a serial philanderer. Maria "Ria" Langham had developed a huge crush after seeing him perform onstage in Houston, and she was determined to insert

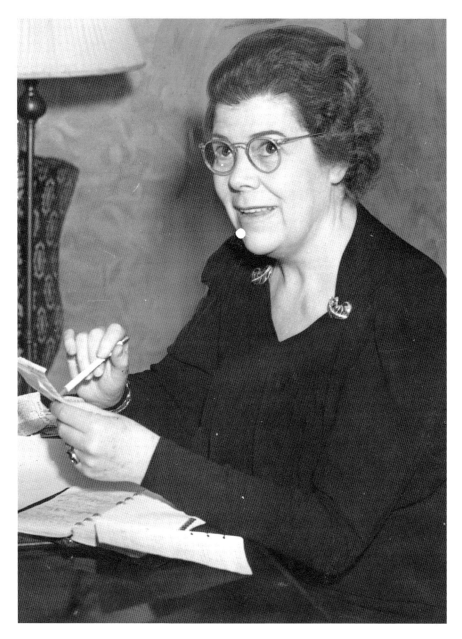

Josephine Dillon as she appeared in 1939, the same year Clark Gable starred in *Gone with the Wind* and married fellow movie star Carole Lombard. It was Josephine's coaching and career guidance that turned Clark Gable into the "King of Hollywood." The problem was that she was seventeen years older than her dashing movie star husband and had a dowdy appearance. *Author's collection.*

herself into his life. Her half brother was also an actor, and he arranged for her to meet Clark Gable backstage in New York.

Like Josephine, Ria was older and worldly. She was also exceptionally wealthy. As their relationship grew, Ria's increasing possessiveness of Clark applied pressure for him to leave Josephine.

As soon as Clark and Josephine's divorce was finalized in 1930, Ria badgered him on the topic of marrying her. She even went so far as to disclose to MGM executives that she and Clark had been living together without benefit of marriage, which directly violated the morality clause in his contract. If they didn't marry, she informed them, there would be no choice but to tell the press about their living arrangement. Clark Gable was now worth a tremendous amount of money to MGM, and they couldn't risk losing their investment. MGM management informed Clark that he had no choice but to marry Ria Langham. They were wed on June 19, 1931.

Meanwhile, Josephine Dillon did not go away quietly. She believed the distinction of being Clark Gable's spurned wife hurt her reputation, and she, too, went directly to MGM to help fix the problem. Without consulting its star, MGM determined that money would be directly deducted from Clark Gable's paycheck to support his ex-wife. He was livid. Clark's humble childhood had another lasting impact on him: he was extremely frugal with his money.

Josephine continued to teach acting, but the cloud of being "Clark Gable's ex-wife" hung over her head. As it turns out, Josephine was correct when she said that marriage to Clark Gable had hurt her once-successful acting coach career. With every career milestone or whenever she would guest lecture at an acting school, newspapers inevitably referred to her as Clark Gable's former wife and acting coach.

In the 1950s, she said, "People will come to me and they will shake their heads and say, 'You poor, poor dear. Isn't it awful how that man Gable treats his wives.' Well, if there was anything wrong with a man, you wouldn't stay for seven years with him."

After Clark's death in 1960, she said in a 1961 newspaper interview that people had called her acting school only to say abusive things to her. Clark Gable biographers were also continually asking her to say terrible things about him for their books or hoping for an inside scoop. She said:

> *I don't know why people think of me unkindly. Just the same a lot of people say they've read about me in these new books and feel they should abuse me. Maybe it is a pathetic jealousy of anyone connected with a popular*

man like Gable….It has been worse since his death. They want me to say
something unflattering or sensational about Clark. They want dirt. But I
continue to refuse to say anything about him for a few dirty dollars. I was
his wife for 10 years, and I can't think of anything belittling about Clark.
And I see no reason for defaming his good name.

She also spoke somewhat kindly about the choices in women he made
after her. "Clark always tried to find a companion," she said. "Too often the
women he knew simply wanted him to get them in the movies. But he was
always very kind. And I am very proud of him and what he stood for. He
always behaved well. It is a difficult thing for a poor boy to have the world's
riches thrust upon him and still be able to keep his balance and ideals. It
takes an extremely strong character. Clark was strong that way."

In that same interview, she also noted that she had never remarried. "I
thought about it several times, but I also thought how unfair it would be to
any man to go through life known as the fellow who married Clark Gable's
first wife."

Likewise, Clark seemed to remember his first wife fondly. As early as 1932,
just a year after marrying his second wife, Ria, Clark said of Josephine, "To
her I owe a great deal of gratitude." Indeed, Josephine is the only former
wife whom Clark remembered in his will, which read:

> *I give, devise and bequeath to JOSEPHINE DILLON, my former wife,*
> *that certain real property situate in the County of Los Angeles, State of*
> *California, known as 12746 Landale, North Hollywood, California, and*
> *more particularly described as follows:*
>   *The West fifty (50) feet of the East one hundred (100) feet of Lot 9,*
> *Tract 5588, as per map recorded in Book 59, page 49, of Maps, in the*
> *office of the Recorder of said County.*

Josephine continued to live in her home until illness prevented her from
living alone. She moved to Rockhaven, where she died on November 11,
1971, after "a long illness." The illness was not disclosed.

Her obituary, which appeared on November 16 in the *Long Beach Independent*,
read, "At 87, Josephine Dillon died last week in a Glendale sanitarium. She
took with her the memory of being the first of Gable's five wives and the one
who saw the golden star over the shoulder of the young roughneck."

CLARK'S NEXT CHAPTER

When Clark Gable married Maria "Ria" Langham in 1931, she was considered one of the wealthiest women in Houston. Her second husband, who had been considerably older than she, left her a fortune when he died. Clark was her fourth husband, and this time, she was the considerably older spouse by seventeen years. He was thirty and she was forty-seven when they married. She was thrilled with the idea of being Mrs. Clark Gable. During their marriage, Clark won his only Academy Award for the movie *It Happened One Night*, and he walked Ria's daughter down the aisle when she got married.

But if Ria was expecting a story that ended happily ever after with her movie star husband, her hopes were soon dashed. Although she lavished Clark with gifts and fine clothing, he started affairs with younger and more glamorous costars, such as Joan Crawford and Loretta Young, with whom he secretly fathered a child. (This secret would not be revealed until decades later.) They also kept separate bedrooms and, eventually, separate homes. The longer they were married, the more Clark distanced himself from his wife.

When Clark danced with actress Carole Lombard at a party in 1936, his marriage to Ria was already in shambles and, as far as he was concerned, practically over. Clark and Carole had starred in a movie called *No Man of Her Own* in 1932, but at the time she was married to William Powell and he was newly married to Ria. No sparks flew on the set in 1932, but that all changed in 1936 when they met again.

Carole was a very different kind of woman from her predecessors in Clark Gable's life. Josephine and Ria had both been significantly older than Clark and were women from whom he could benefit. Carole Lombard was his equal. Like Clark Gable, she was glamorous and a highly paid movie star. She was also more age appropriate, as she was seven years younger than Clark. Ria had held out hope that Clark would return to her, just as he had after his other affairs. But he was besotted with Carole and wanted to marry her. Clark divorced Ria and married Carole Lombard in March 1939 during a weekend off from shooting *Gone with the Wind*.

The marriage was happy but didn't last. On the evening of January 16, 1942, an airplane carrying Carole Lombard; her mother, Bess Peters; and MGM press agent (and one of Clark's closest friends) Otto Winkler crashed into the side of Potosi Mountain in the Nevada desert. The plane had

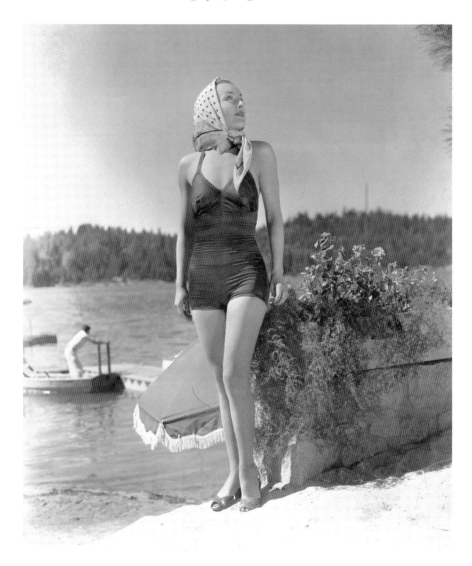

Carole Lombard at the height of her movie stardom. Her tragic death left her widower, Clark Gable, devastated for years. It was likely his depression and a need to find another version of Carole that inspired him to marry Lady Sylvia Ashley. *Author's collection.*

refueled just outside Las Vegas and crashed thirteen minutes after takeoff. All twenty-two passengers were killed instantly.

By all accounts, Clark Gable never fully recovered from Carole Lombard's death. A few years later, he was still deeply grieving. He dated a few women but was especially vulnerable when he encountered a charming former showgirl from London. That showgirl had an equally charming socialite sister who eventually retired at Rockhaven. The sisters' lives were incredibly entwined, and both aimed to better their circumstances through connections in Hollywood.

Enter Lady Sylvia Ashley

Lady Sylvia Ashley married Clark Gable in 1949, only to find herself divorced from him sixteen months later. Those closest to Clark said he confided to friends within weeks of their marriage that he had made a mistake in marrying the former showgirl. Sylvia appeared devastated by the end of her time with Clark.

Lady Ashley had been married first to British aristocracy, which is how she got the title "Lady," and then to film royalty Douglas Fairbanks Sr., the silent movie star who held the title of the "King of Hollywood" before Clark Gable later inherited the nickname. Sylvia found herself on the receiving end of considerable ire when Fairbanks left his wife and business partner, Mary Pickford, for her. Doug and Sylvia were married until his death in 1939, but the public blamed her for the breakup of Hollywood's first power couple and never really forgot or forgave her.

When Clark and Sylvia began dating, no one took the relationship seriously; Clark was still dating other women. But something somewhere happened between them, because the pair married in a friend's living room on December 20, 1949. Sylvia's sister, Vera Bleck, served as matron of honor, and her husband, British film producer Basil Bleck, gave the bride away. Even close friends were surprised by the wedding and exclaimed, "*Who?*" when it was learned that Clark had once again tied the knot.

The marriage was rocky from the start. The only explanation friends could come up with for the relationship was Sylvia's vague resemblance to Carole Lombard. Clark and Sylvia were different on a fundamental level. Clark was a rugged outdoorsman and Sylvia loved antiques and large social events. Clark, notoriously tight with a dollar, was appalled by Sylvia's extravagant spending. Another bone of contention was her nephew Timothy, whom she spoiled with gifts and money to travel. Her fondness for her sister's children was even noted by syndicated newspaper columnist Sheila Graham. "'She adores children,' I am told by Sylvia's best friend in Hollywood—Agent Minna Wallis. 'Sylvia just can't do enough for her

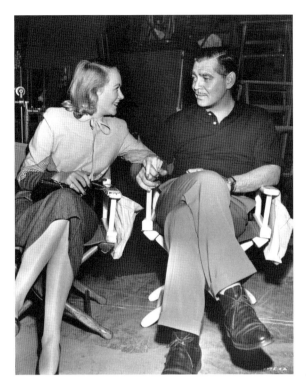

Sylvia Gable visits her new husband, Clark Gable, on the set of *To Please a Lady* in 1950. The marriage between Clark and Sylvia began deteriorating almost immediately after their December 1949 wedding. Sylvia and her sister Vera Bleck, who retired to Rockhaven, were working-class women who married into the Hollywood elite. Few people in Clark's inner circle understood his attraction to Sylvia, other than her passing resemblance to his former wife Carole Lombard, who died in a 1942 plane crash. *Author's collection.*

nephew and niece (Timothy, 17, and Loretta, 14) son and daughter of her sister Vera Bleck." Timothy was so entitled that he took to borrowing money from MGM, which Uncle Clark was then obligated to pay back.

Just as he had done years earlier with Ria, Clark began shutting down and distancing himself from his wife. He also began drinking heavily, to the point friends noticed his despair. When he finally announced to Sylvia that he wanted a divorce, she thought he was joking and stayed in the house—the same house that Clark had shared with Carole. But Clark grew increasingly sullen and silent in her presence. When it was clear that Clark wasn't joking about a divorce and he had no intention of changing his opinion, Sylvia finally moved out.

As soon as she was gone, Clark started erasing any evidence Sylvia had ever lived on his ranch. He removed her belongings, changed the locks and fired her staff. His behavior after their separation no doubt stung. Sylvia gave in and filed for divorce in May 1951 and went back to her former name, Lady Sylvia Ashley. Newspapers were already reporting that Clark's marriage to Sylvia had been a mistake, a shadow that hung over her name for the rest of her life. Sylvia's reputation already had negative connotations because she was "the other woman" who came between Douglas Fairbanks Sr. and Mary Pickford. Now she had the misfortune of following in Carole Lombard's footsteps and was labeled a "mistake."

Sylvia was devastated. Days after filing for divorce, she boarded a ship for a cruise around the South Seas. Newspapers reported that doctors advised her to take a lengthy rest. Brother-in-law Basil Bleck told newspaper reporters she was close to a nervous breakdown. It was Vera and Basil who supported Sylvia both publicly and privately while she began the process of rebuilding her life after Clark Gable and her breakdown.

Sylvia went on to remarry (this time to a Georgian prince) and found happiness in the marriage, which lasted until her death in 1977. A section of the *Valley Times* newspaper called Media Meow reported her death in September. "The *Times*, that bastion of the obituary, finally got around to telling its readers that Lady Sylvia Ashley died on June 30 in L.A. of cancer at age 73. (She'd been wed to Doug Fairbanks Sr. and Clark Gable, among others)....P.S. Her sister Vera Bleck was so distraught when Sylvia died that she did not make the death known publicly."

The sisters had always been close, and together the British-born women enjoyed the lives of Hollywood socialites. Sylvia's name was connected with considerably bigger names and scandal because of her marriages to both Hollywood "kings," but both sisters traveled in elite circles. (In 1941, they even founded the British Distressed Areas Fund with actress Constance Bennett and Virginia Fox Zanuck, wife of Twentieth Century Fox studio head Darryl Zanuck, to help World War II refugees.)

Vera outlived her sister by almost twenty years and spent her retirement at Rockhaven, where her children visited her. She passed away on January 1, 1997. The sisters who rose from working-class origins in England to a life of glamour in Hollywood are still together. Both are buried (fittingly) at Hollywood Forever Cemetery in Los Angeles.

Chapter 7

Noteworthy Residents of Rockhaven

During seventy years of operation, hundreds of women found safety and rest on the grounds of Rockhaven Sanitarium. Each was unique and had her own story, but some women were especially noteworthy. Here's a small sampling of the women of Rockhaven.

FEARLESS PEGGY FEARS

Peggy Fears was more than just a pretty face. The showgirl turned producer turned entrepreneur lived a life worthy of the movies or a Broadway production. Born on June 1, 1903, in New Orleans to a banker father, Peggy later moved with her family to Dallas, Texas, during her youth. Against her father's wishes, she left home at sixteen with the desire to be a star of the stage. From the very beginning, Peggy Fears was a force to be reckoned with.

While living in New York, Peggy went on a date with Yale student Jock Whitney of the famed Whitney family. Jock had an interest in the performing arts and later went on to invest in Broadway plays, found Pioneer Pictures, help fund *Gone with the Wind* and serve as president of the Museum of Modern Art. Their date at the Richman Club turned out to be a pivotal night in Peggy's young life. During an evening filled with dancing and singing, singer and actress Helen Morgan overheard Peggy crooning a song and told her, "Kid, you're ripe for Ziegfeld."

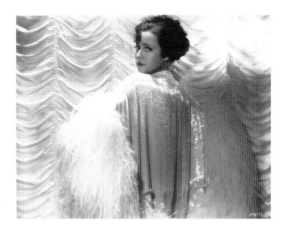

Peggy Fears was as smart as she was beautiful. She came from a typical middle-class upbringing and turned herself into a Ziegfeld Follies dancer, successful theater producer, nightclub act and resort entrepreneur. *Author's collection.*

Peggy took the suggestion seriously and soon landed herself an audition with Florenz "Flo" Ziegfeld, producer of the lavish Ziegfeld Follies. She landed a job, and in her first Ziegfeld production, *No Foolin'*, she worked in the chorus line alongside other future stars Paulette Goddard, Susan Fleming, Claire Luce and Baby Vogt. It wasn't long before Peggy was rubbing elbows with other stars in New York. Peggy, a bisexual, began a romantic relationship with actress Louise Brooks, who later wrote about the affair in her autobiography, *Lulu in Hollywood*. Louise wrote that she never allowed the relationship to get too serious (at least as far as she was concerned) and that the two young women were friends with fellow performer W.C. Fields and sometimes visited him in his dressing room backstage.

In the late 1920s, Peggy married A.C. Blumenthal ("Blumey"), a wealthy man involved in real estate and theater. Together, the couple began producing plays on Broadway and, within the first three years of their marriage, made $15 million.

In 1932, Congress summoned several noteworthy Broadway producers to speak at a meeting regarding theater critics and their habits. Peggy Fears was successful enough to receive an invitation and, in fact, the only producer to accept. Peggy traveled to Washington, D.C., where she was asked if critics were responsible for the economic depression theaters were currently experiencing. A newspaper reported, "She replied by asking them if they would say that just because a story appeared in the newspapers that stocks had gone down again, whether these newspapers could be blamed for the stock market crash."

The newspaper further praised Peggy for her ability to see both sides of the issue. Although she recommended that critics should make clear that their reviews were opinions, she also noted that their function was necessary.

"No art has been able to exist without criticism," she told Congress. "The theater is no exception. There must be critics to guide the public and to establish a standard of excellence and good taste for the producers to follow. I have no fight with the critics. On the contrary, I am grateful to them."

Peggy also received compliments for actually attending the congressional meeting when no other producers or theater managers did. As it was reported, "Where some of the other managers, who would like to have their say about the critics, contented themselves with penning sugared and secret notes to Congressman [William Irving] Sirovich, it remained for the newest and youngest of them all to exhibit the courage of her convictions. The other managers, perhaps were afraid that if they spoke their mind, the critics, like elephants, would not forget and take pleasure in belaboring future offerings from their productorial steliers. Miss Fears, with the desire to be fair to both the reviewers and the theater, did what she thought was right."

Peggy and Blumey were more than just respected in their line of work. Their productions brought in millions, but they spent almost as much as they earned. They lived lavishly in a Manhattan penthouse, and Peggy owned five Rolls-Royces and a $65,000 chinchilla coat. Meanwhile, their fortune dwindled to just $300 in savings.

The marriage was as stormy as their finances. Blumey was often jealous when photographers shoved him aside to get pictures of his beautiful wife. They weathered an involuntary bankruptcy against a dress shop she owned. Peggy continued touring with her nightclub singing act to earn money. They fought constantly, separated in 1934 and then reconciled.

The pair separated yet again in 1936 when Peggy spent six weeks in Jamaica. Upon her return to the United States, she threatened her husband that this latest separation would become a divorce unless he paid $55,000 in back alimony. She also announced she would also seek a court order to confiscate his property. That wasn't all. Peggy further argued that she was owed $40,000 in alimony from their 1934 separation agreement. Blumey countered that she had violated the terms of their agreement by moving into New York's Ambassador Hotel, where he lived. According to their formal legal separation, Peggy was not permitted live in the same building where her husband resided. Meanwhile, Blumey had hired private detectives to follow his wife and had her telephone line tapped. Somehow, the couple managed to resolve their differences. In 1939, a newspaper reported that Peggy and Blumey had reconciled yet again and were living on Sunset Boulevard in Hollywood. Later, they moved into a large mansion in the Larchmont neighborhood, but the house burned to the ground. The road was never smooth for the marriage. They separated and reconciled multiple times, including going so far as to renew their vows at certain points. All totaled, the couple had three wedding ceremonies during their relationship.

Her turbulent marriage wasn't the only difficulty she experienced during this time. In 1939, Peggy's mother committed suicide at the age of fifty-four by turning on the gas in her Dallas home. Peggy's father, Edgar, found the body when he returned home from work and told authorities that his wife had been ill for some time.

It is unclear if her marriage brought her any comfort after her mother's suicide. Peggy sued for a formal separation and alimony in 1945, only for the pair to again reconcile. But it was not to last. They separated for good in 1950, and by this time, Peggy was forty-nine (though she probably claimed younger) and in need of reinventing herself. Though living again in Manhattan, she visited Fire Island in 1952 and, during her stay, purchased some property after a friend's suggestion. Initially, however, she was unimpressed with the Long Island beach community. "Actually, I loathe sand and I hate the ocean," she said. "Anyway, I was very happy sunbathing on my terrace in New York. I had the most marvelous penthouse. Fire Island was so far to go for one day, but one weekend in 1952 I went with friends to Point O Woods. So dull. You can't drink, and you must put on a dress for dinner, but who wants to be in Ocean Beach in the middle of the season?"

After purchasing her property, Peggy continued her singing career, touring London and Paris for three years. When she returned to New York, friends encouraged her to build on her land. The result was the Pines Yacht Club, hotel and restaurant on the water where guests could park their boats. The advertisements called it a "botel." She also built a private residence for herself, and soon her show business friends were showing up at Peggy's resort. It also began attracting other wealthy and artistic guests, such as fashion models, producers, writers and stockbrokers. "I want it to be a little like the Riviera," she said in 1960, also noting that the area was attracting big names like Marlene Dietrich, Marilyn Monroe, Polly Bergen, Ella Logan, Martha Raye and Tennessee Williams.

Around this time, Peggy found love once again. Tedi Thurman was a statuesque redheaded model, radio personality and actress who is best remembered as Miss Monitor, the sultry "weather girl" who gave weather reports on NBC from 1955 to 1961. She appeared on the original *Tonight Show* with Jack Paar in 1957, and *TV Guide* even featured an article about her called "Tedi Thurman: Weathergirl Supreme." Tedi and Peggy became friends and, according to Tedi, found they had so much in common that

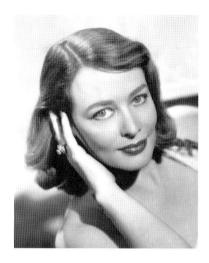

Statuesque redhead Tedi Thurman became Peggy's companion from the 1950s until Peggy was hospitalized at Rockhaven. It is said that Tedi continued to visit Peggy at Rockhaven, even though she had moved to Palm Springs.

they took their relationship further. It was a partnership that lasted "until she had to be hospitalized," Tedi said later in an interview. That is, the relationship lasted decades until Peggy moved to Rockhaven.

In 1958, a call from Los Angeles informed Peggy that Blumey was now dying after a heart attack. She flew west to be by his side in California. Her former husband, with whom she had made millions of dollars, died broke.

More bad news was coming. In 1959, a fire broke out at Peggy's resort. No one was hurt, and the guests were able to evacuate their boats to safety, but the property was destroyed. "In less than an hour and a half, nothing was left," Peggy said. "Not even my beautiful trees. Thank God no one was hurt. Yes, that Sunday morning was my birthday. Naturally, all those beautiful birthday presents everyone brought me were gone; but they all said immediately that I must build something new and right then my designer friend Luis Estevez did this marvelous sketch. Modern as could be. He never left my side through all of it."

Peggy kept her word to rebuild the resort. This time, much of the structure was built with aluminum as a fire prevention. Under her stern direction, the new building went up in almost record time. She ran the property until 1966, when she sold it to former male model John Whyte. It was under Whyte's ownership that Peggy's resort and Fire Island became known as a haven for the LGBT community.

After selling her resort, Peggy found herself living a relatively quiet life in California, but she still participated in the occasional project. In 1970, for instance, Peggy was offered a technical advisor role for Hal Prince's show *Follies*.

By the 1980s, Peggy was showing signs of dementia and, at some point during the decade, came to live at Rockhaven Sanitarium for the remainder of her senior years. Tedi Thurman, who resided in Palm Springs, continued to visit her at Rockhaven. Rockhaven's staff enjoyed dressing Peggy up "like a doll" as a tribute to her glamorous youth. Dementia crippled Peggy, who had once been so tenacious and brilliant. As with many dementia patients, speaking became increasingly difficult and, consequently, rare. The woman who had sung for audiences and spoken before Congress was now robbed of her ability to speak. Nurses sometimes played old records of Peggy singing so she could listen to her younger self. The kind gesture reinvigorated Peggy and occasionally stimulated not only her memory but her dormant vocal cords as well. During these times, Peggy sometimes perked up and exclaimed, "That's me!"

Peggy Fears died peacefully on August 24, 1994, at Rockhaven.

Gwen Lee: The Beautiful Flapper

Like a lot of actresses working in the late 1920s and early 1930s, Gwen Lee fashioned herself in the image of an effervescent flapper. She enjoyed modest to decent success on the stage and in movies, but her career began to fizzle by the '30s. Some of that was the rotten luck and fierce competition that can come when gambling on a career in Hollywood. However, her career was also damaged by a lawsuit filed against her by her own mother, who charged that Gwen was mentally unstable and in need of a conservator. The lawsuit resulted in a brief stay at Rockhaven, and Gwen earns the dubious distinction of being one of the few women who was possibly placed there on trumped-up allegations. It's tough to tell what the truth is, but Gwen's family was troubled from her earliest years.

Gwendolyn Lepinski was born on November 14, 1904, in Hastings, Nebraska, to a barber father and hairdresser mother. The Lepinski family faced some serious challenges during Gwen's youth. Her father, Frank, was a veteran of the Spanish-American War, and it appears he developed a drinking problem that caused stress in his marriage. Gwen's mother, Mriette (who went by Etta), actually sued "A.L. Yarter (et al)" for $15,000 in damages for selling her husband alcohol. On January 5, 1910, it was reported that the lawsuit had been settled after Yarter agreed to pay $600 and court costs.

More upheaval came in August when fire destroyed the Adroit hairdressing parlor that Etta owned. The building was a total loss and only partially covered by insurance. Worse, two firemen sustained injuries from falling glass while fighting the blaze. It was determined that the fire was started by a gas jet in the workroom.

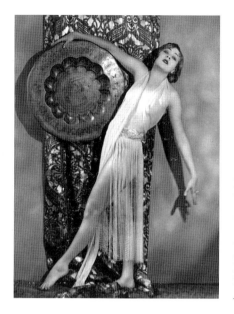

Actress Gwen Lee looked like she was poised for stardom in Hollywood, but fate dealt her a terrible blow. Thanks to her mother's accusations of mental instability, Gwen briefly stayed at Rockhaven in the early 1930s. It remains one of the few cases in which a woman may have gone to Rockhaven on false charges. The scandal hurt Gwen's career, and it never recovered. *Author's collection.*

But the worst was yet to come. By early 1911, Etta decided she'd had enough of her husband's alcoholism and made an unusual move for the era when she filed for divorce on the grounds of cruelty, drunkenness and nonsupport. Not long after, she left for California. Frank was devastated and brooded over the loss of his family for the next three months. He committed suicide at the age of thirty-four in April 1911 when his daughter was just six years old. He shot himself in the temple in a shoe shop owned by his father, Anton Lepinski. The *Nebraska State Journal* reported on April 16, 1911, "About a month ago Mrs. Lepinski and her brother went to California to live and it is thought that her departure with their child caused him to kill himself."

It is not known how long Etta was in California, but records indicate she was back in Nebraska by at least 1916. The 1920 census indicates that Etta was living with her fifteen-year-old daughter and her sixty-two-year-mother, Loretta Kennedy, in Scotts Bluff, Nebraska. (Interestingly, Etta did not list herself as divorced but as "widowed" on the census report, so the divorce probably wasn't finalized when Frank died.) Gwendolyn, meanwhile, was growing into a lovely young woman and began modeling clothes at department stores. She was discovered by Monta Bell, a director, producer and screenwriter, who saw potential in this youngster from Nebraska.

Gwendolyn Lepinski was renamed Gwen Lee and moved to Los Angeles. In 1923, her name appears in the *Los Angeles Times* as part of the Prudent

Prue and Patient Peggy Club, which was formed by a group of "Hollywood Beauties" who were focusing their time and energy on self-betterment and culture. The club emphasized the importance of modest dress, listening to directors' instructions, not kissing members of the opposite sex (unless for a scene on camera), not talking or laughing too loudly in public and not chewing gum or smoking. The article also mentions that the young women had all been recently signed to contracts with Preferred Pictures. The studio most likely planted the article to emphasize what proper young ladies it had working in its movies.

The following year, Gwen's career was picking up steam, and Preferred Pictures promoted her as one of the twelve most beautiful girls in Hollywood. As her profile increased, her name and photo appeared in newspapers more often, talking about things like what she was wearing, what she liked to do in her spare time (swimming and going to the beach) and her upcoming movie roles. In 1925, her movie career received a boost by signing with Metro-Goldwyn-Mayer, a considerably larger studio than Preferred. The *Lincoln Star* reported about the local girl making it big in Hollywood: "Director Hobart Henley picked Gwen Lee out of the extra ranks and snatched her up for Metro—statuesque, blonde, beautiful—what more can you ask?" Gwen was moving from extra and starlet to "latest blonde" status. She began playing mostly secondary roles, but her costars were such names as Norma Shearer, Billie Dove and the ultimate 1920s flapper of the silent era, Clara Bow. Her costars' noteworthy names indicate the high caliber of the movies she was appearing in.

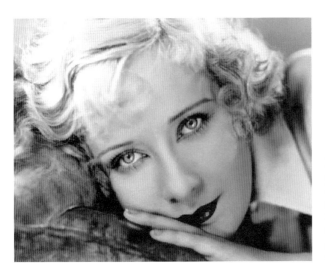

In the 1920s and early 1930s, Gwen Lee worked steadily as an actress and was considered one of the movie industry's great beauties. *Author's collection.*

She worked constantly and made nearly forty movies between the years 1925 and 1930 alone. When not on a movie set, she was starring in productions at night in the theater. In 1928, she was named one of the WAMPAS Baby Stars, an honor bestowed by the United States Western Association of Motion Pictures Advertisers to young women believed to be on the threshold of major stardom. As movies made the slow transition from silent to sound, Gwen was one of the fortunate actors whose speaking voice was deemed attractive enough for the new technology. Countless other talented actors weren't as lucky, and their careers died almost overnight.

It seemed as though Gwen was destined for major stardom. She was receiving regular, positive coverage in the press. She was starring alongside the box office's most famous stars. She had made the dreaded transition from silent movies. She worked for a top studio. And yet, Gwen's career stalled. For as well as things were going, her career never moved beyond to that final step of stardom: leading lady roles. During the Great Depression, studios began scaling back the number of actors and actresses on contract. Contract or stock players, as they were called, were paid weekly salaries regardless of whether they worked. Such a system was no longer sustainable, so studios started releasing many actors from their contracts, and in 1931, Gwen Lee was one of them. She continued working on a freelance basis, but her days of a secure weekly salary were over. It was very poor timing.

Sometime around late 1931 or early 1932, Etta Lepinski made accusations that her daughter was mentally unstable and incompetent to handle her own affairs. That claim turned into a lawsuit in March 1932 when Etta formally sued Gwen to seek control over her daughter's personal property and jewelry, which were valued at $1,000. The *Chicago Tribune* reported on March 14 that Gwen "recorded a horrified protest over an action filed by her mother, Mrs. Etta Lepinski." The short article closed with an unusual comment by Gwen's lawyer: "The suit won't stay on the court files long, according to Thomas Higgin, attorney for the actress, who said the mother and daughter have patched up their differences."

This cryptic statement begs the question: what, exactly, were their "differences"?

It was around this time that Gwen found herself at Rockhaven Sanitarium. Though it had been open for less than ten years, Rockhaven was already enjoying a reputation for high-quality mental healthcare. It was also geographically close to Hollywood, so if Gwen was in need of mental health assistance, Rockhaven would have been an ideal placement for her. But was she really in need of help? According to Crescenta Valley historian and Rockhaven expert Mike Lawler, this is one of the very few cases in which a resident's placement at the sanitarium can be called into question. It will never be known at this point, but Thomas Higgin appears to have been correct. The lawsuit did not last, and just a few weeks after making that comment, Etta Lepinski dropped her suit against Gwen.

The *Los Angeles Times* reported on April 1 that Etta Lepinski had dropped the incompetency charges against her daughter, as her health was "much improved." Etta's attorney, C.C. Caswell, was quoted as saying that it was Gwen—not Etta—who had asked that her mother be appointed guardian over her property, which is in contrast to the report in March that Gwen was "horrified" by the lawsuit.

Although her mother's lawsuit was dropped, the scandal damaged Gwen's career. Whether or not Gwen had been ill almost didn't matter; the public believed she had been. Etta had told newspapers that Gwen had *regained* her health. After the suit was dismissed, newspapers reported, "Gwen Lee, blond Polish girl, was one of the most popular actresses on the MGM contract list for several years until she fell into ill health."

That story, however, can't possibly be true because Gwen's contract was not renewed along with multiple others when MGM let several actors go to save money, as reported in newspapers the *year before* in July 1931:

> The practice of carrying large numbers of players on long-term contracts and medium salaries is fast dying out in Hollywood. There is a tendency to reach out and get the player for the role regardless of their affiliation. When M.G.M. released Gwen Lee, for instance, from one of those stock contracts which had kept her tied to the lot, although without a role for the major portion of the final year of her service, they discovered that she was ideal for a role in a picture they were casting. Gwen Lee was called back to the lot which had just found no need for her services as a stock player and given an excellent part. Gwen Lee now is a free-lance player of opportunity to do the type thing for which she is eminently fitted.

Gwen's career slowed down significantly after the scandal surrounding her mental health. Later that year, in October 1932, Gwen's name again made the newspapers for the wrong reasons when she was named as a defendant in a lawsuit for not paying a clothing bill. The New York Cloak and Suit house sued Gwen for $411. It's impossible to know why Gwen was behind in her bills. Was it because work was harder to come by? Did she really have mental health issues? Was someone else responsible for paying her bills? Had she simply forgotten? Regardless of the reason, it was more negative publicity.

Gwen continued to work in theater and movies, but her career in motion pictures was over by 1938. Very little is known of Gwen after 1938 other than she married a man named George Mence Jr. on May 4, 1943, in California. She eventually left California, but she fell off the radar after that. She died in Reno, Nevada, on August 20, 1961, at the age of fifty-six. She had appeared in more than sixty films during her career but was mostly forgotten by the time of her death.

Babe Egan, the Hollywood Redhead

Babe Egan was a violinist and bandleader during the Jazz Age. What was unique about her band was that she was a female bandleader in charge of an all-woman band. Babe Egan and the Hollywood Redheads, as they were called, were a pioneering musical act.

Mary Florence "Babe" Egan was the youngest of seven children born in Seattle in 1897 or 1900 (depending on the source) to Jack Egan, a newspaper reporter, and Alice Doran Egan. Both parents were of Irish descent and Catholic.

Babe came to Los Angeles with her widowed mother and a brother and, according to the 1920 census, worked as a professional violinist. In a 1974 interview with Babe's former drummer and family friend, Estelle "Stell" Dilthey said Babe earned a living playing background music for silent movies in Hollywood movie theaters but longed for her own band. Stell, who came from a musical family, eventually joined the band Babe was so determined to create. "Babe just went around finding the youngest, cleanest cut, best young girl musicians in Los Angeles," said Stell, whose sister Elva also joined the band for about a year. "I had practically no competition on drums."

Being an all-girl band was enough of a gimmick to garner attention, but they had something else going for them: all the women had red hair. Babe, a natural redhead, called her outfit Babe Egan and the Hollywood Redheads (sometimes billed Hollywood Red Heads). Only three of the women in the band, however, naturally had red hair. The rest wore bobbed red wigs. Their first performance was at the Sacramento Fair, probably in 1924. Eventually, they began booking better gigs, including theater openings, the first of which was on June 17, 1925, at the Hollywood Ravenna Theatre. "We'd start playing at the beginning of the picture, and then we'd play for the newsreel," Stell recalled. "Then the big Wurlitzer pipe organ would take over while we prepared for our act on stage."

The girls each earned sixty-five dollars per week. They owned their instruments, and Babe provided the outfits. "We wore blue and white striped blazers, the collegiate look," Stell said. "It was a sort of all-American girl act in which we all did a little bit of everything."

In early 1925, Babe's band was hitting the theater and vaudeville circuit and, by December, had sailed the Pacific to perform in Hawaii, where they played for twelve weeks "to packed houses." Other engagements followed, including several weeks at home in Los Angeles, a week in Denver and a summer in Chicago. The Redheads were booked at the Rialto Theater in Casper, Wyoming, and the local newspaper touted, "Their engagement here is a part of the program of the Rialto to have high class added attractions."

As the Redheads toured the United States, they gained a reputation not only for their red hair and beauty but also for actually having talent and putting on a good show. A Pennsylvania newspaper said in 1926:

> *Under the direction of Babe Egan they supply a program that at no time is permitted to even lag or smack of a sameness that oft-times proves uninteresting. On the other hand these girls give enough variety to compel admiration as well as appreciation. Not only do they contribute a most satisfying number of syncopated melodies on various instruments but intersperse their efforts either with songs or dances and here and there a solo number introduced that appeals to patrons in every part of the theatre.*

By 1928, it was said that Babe was the highest-paid woman on vaudeville's Orpheum Theater circuit. That year, she purchased her own house in the Los Angeles suburb of Van Nuys, though she wasn't home very often. For the next few years, the group toured almost constantly. They crisscrossed the United States, and their reputation was such that the *Akron Beacon Journal* praised them as "one of vaudeville's best known jazz bands."

After experiencing a huge amount of success on American stages, Babe and her Redheads traveled to Canada and Europe. The group returned home to America triumphant and continued their rigorous touring schedule. On occasion, actress and radio personality Thelma White joined them onstage to sing. By 1934, the group was appearing under different names, such as Babe Egan and her Orchestra, Babe Egan and her Debutantes, Miss

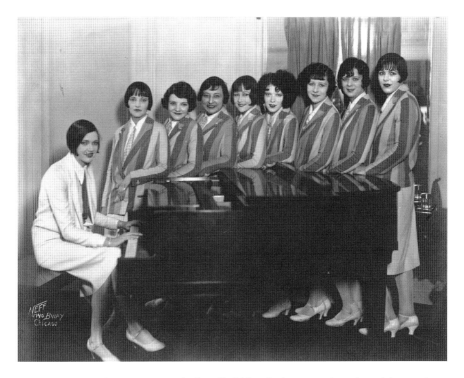

Babe Egan selected young women for her all-girl band who were talented musicians and "clean cut." Babe supplied the collegiate-style blazers, and the women used their own instruments. Babe Egan and her Hollywood Redheads were a huge hit on the vaudeville circuit.

Egan and her All-Girl Band and Babe Egan and her Modern Continentals. It seemed like every new stop garnered a new name. Thelma White was also frequently included on the bill.

For as much success as Babe and her group had in the 1920s and the first half of the 1930s, jobs were drying up for them by the middle of the decade. Babe's name appeared in the *Los Angeles Times* in 1936, but not for a gig—she attended a costume party thrown by Mary Louis Emmet in honor of Collete Bertram, a woman from New York.

Musical appearances were almost nonexistent, although Hedda Hopper did report in 1942 that her assistant managed to gather up some acts to entertain soldiers in Mojave, Babe Egan and her orchestra among them. Mostly, when her name appeared in the newspaper it was for her personal life. For instance, she served as maid of honor for her niece, actress Betty Harron, when she married a Hollywood studio makeup man, Ern Westmore, at 460 South Las Palmas in Los Angeles in February 1941. In 1943, her

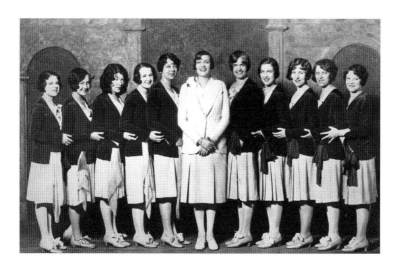

Mary Florence Egan, nicknamed "Babe," was the youngest of seven children born to an Irish American family. From early on, she was a gifted musician. She was also a natural redhead and, when possible, tried to hire other redheads for her band. When needed, women with different-colored hair wore red wigs so Babe could continue calling her band "the Hollywood Redheads."

sister, Elizabeth Beckwith, passed away in Seattle, and "Miss Babe Egan of Hollywood" was listed as one of her survivors.

Her career as a handsomely paid musician had come to an end. All-girl bands, no matter how talented, were no longer in demand. Newspaper columnist Hugh Dixon reported in 1944, "Babe Egan, whose Hollywood Red-Heads was the first of the big-time all-girl bands, is now a wardrobe mistress at RKO." Babe continued in the wardrobe department for the next several years. After having a stroke, she could no longer live on her own and moved to Rockhaven, where relatives paid for her stay.

Like many who have had strokes, Babe had aphasia, which made it difficult for her to speak or for others to understand her. The condition didn't stop her from accepting visitors, including family and former band members, and from exchanging letters with friends. Her mobility was affected somewhat, and at one point during her stay at Rockhaven, she fell and broke a hip.

Babe lived at Rockhaven for the last few years of her life, until she passed away on February 7, 1966. The adjustment of going from famous bandleader to wardrobe mistress to stroke victim was difficult for Babe. Thelma White, who visited her old friend from the music circuit, believed Babe was lonely in her final years and living in the past. "People forget you when you get older," she told Thelma.

RAGDOLL DANCER MARION STADLER

The vaudeville era was filled with countless musical, dance and comedy acts. Sometimes those disciplines crossed over, as it did in the case of Don Rose and Marion Stadler, who delighted audiences with their comedy and dance routines.

Marion Eleanor Stadler was born in 1911 in Glendale, California, to Harold and Ella Stadler. Her parents owned a local grocery in the Atwater section of town, and the family lived near their business, along with one of Marion's grandmothers.

From an early age, Marion showed an interest in dance and took lessons while growing up, even giving a ballet performance at her eighth-grade graduation ceremony. Marion's professional dance career began in her teens with a male dance partner, Matt Duffin. The team of Stadler & Duffin only lasted from 1926 to 1927 before the pair went their separate ways.

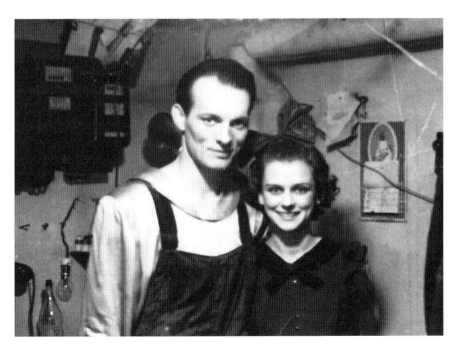

Dance partners—and later married couple—Don Rose and Marion Stadler wowed audiences in the 1930s with their comedic dance routines. The highly athletic act depicted Don trying to dance with a "ragdoll," played by Marion. Their act took them around the world. Here they are pictured backstage waiting to go on at Café Adria in Warsaw in 1935.

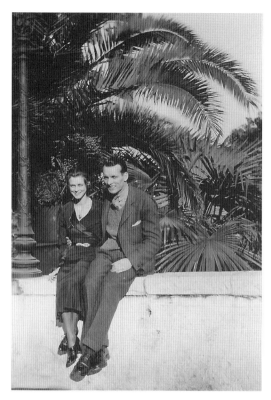

Left: Don and Marion sitting outside their hotel in Monte Carlo on December 29, 1933.

Below: Don and Marion Rose in 1982. They remained a happy and devoted couple until he passed away in 1987.

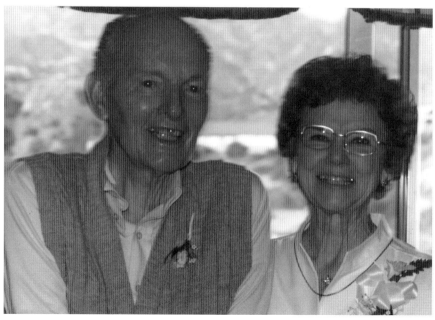

Marion had a new partner by 1928, a young man by the name of Don Rose, who had made a name for himself by dancing without any formal training. He liked to get laughs, and the partnership of Stadler & Rose consisted of Don trying to dance around with a "ragdoll," played by Marion. Their popularity grew to such that they appeared in the 1930 film *The King of Jazz* with Bing Crosby and Paul Whiteman. *The King of Jazz* preserves on film several vaudeville acts, Stadler & Rose's "Ragamuffin Romeo" dance among them.

The duo successfully toured during the 1930s, not just all over America and Canada but in London, Rome, Paris, Havana, Budapest, Copenhagen, Berlin, Mexico City and Rio de Janeiro as well. Their act was a smash hit, and they were asked to perform with Bob Hope, Lawrence Welk and others.

World War II ended their adventures abroad. As it happened, they were appearing in Germany when the war broke out, so the couple was eager to come home to the United States. They made it after several weeks aboard a Danish ship with a red cross painted on the side. After they retired from dancing, the two pursued other careers—together. The dance partners became marriage partners in 1936, and they remained married for fifty-one years, until Don's death on September 4, 1987. Marion lived on her own in their home for the next few years until retiring to Rockhaven in 1994. She was described as a soft-spoken but energetic lady who enjoyed the gardens and daily activities. She also shared a video of her dance routine with friends from the Oaks Cottage at one point. Marion Stadler Rose thrived during her time at Rockhaven. She passed away on December 23, 2001.

THE MOTHER OF MR. JONES

Before there was "Weird" Al Yankovic, there was Spike Jones. Spike made his name thanks to his gift for creating satirical songs, but his love for music started much earlier in childhood.

Lindley Armstrong Jones was born on December 14, 1912, in Long Beach, California, to Lindley Murray Jones, a station agent for Southern Pacific Railroad, and Ada Armstrong Jones, a schoolteacher. The younger Lindley earned the nickname Spike in his youth when he was compared to a railroad spike because of his slender frame.

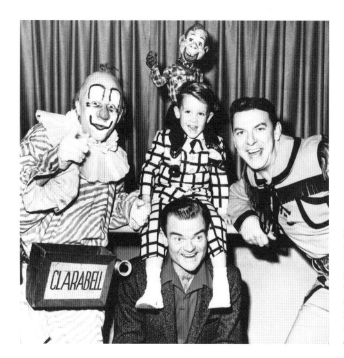

Spike Jones was the equivalent of "Weird Al" Yankovic today. His songs were humorous, and he was just as much a comedian as a musician. *Author's collection.*

Spike showed musical ability from a young age. While attending elementary school, he began playing with the school orchestra, so his parents gifted him with a drum set for Christmas when he was eleven. They had just one rule for him: no jazz! Spike kept up with the instrument, continuing to play in the school orchestra until he graduated from high school and forming his own band, Spike Jones and His Five Tacks. Even while attending junior college, he continued to play with both the school band and around the Los Angeles area.

Spike's persistence in music paid off, and he began landing radio gigs and better jobs with big-name performers in the 1930s. Spike was talented, but he was also bored playing the same songs every night. Inevitably, he put together a group of musicians and began experimenting with satirical material. He struck paydirt in 1942 with "Der Fuehrer's Face," a song ridiculing Adolf Hitler. That song propelled Spike to fame and fortune, and a series of hits parodying popular songs of the day followed.

His musical career flourished, as did another business: sometime around 1949, he opened the Spike Jones Market in La Crescenta. Spike was married to singer Helen Grayco, whose real last name was Greco, a family local to the area. The store was opened with the Greco family in some capacity, either as partners or with Helen's brothers as managers. A Greco

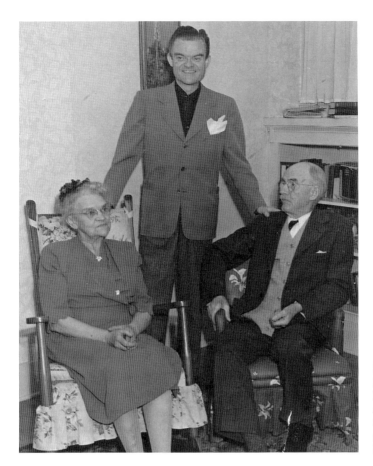

Spike with his parents, Murray and Ada. His mother went on to retire at Rockhaven.

uncle and nephew were also involved. "With all the in-laws I have, I figure I'm good for at least 10 more stores," Spike joked. The supermarket was a fixture in the Valley during the postwar boom and sported a large sign bearing a caricature of the musical comedian.

Spike's financial success allowed him to place his mother, Ada, in Rockhaven when she could no longer care for herself. Spike clearly had ties to the area, as demonstrated by his Spike Jones Market and local in-laws, so he had probably heard about Rockhaven's excellent reputation. Little is known about Ada Jones's stay at Rockhaven, but a photo she had of Spike, his wife, Helen, and their children was found at the sanitarium. Spike had inscribed the photo, "To Mama...."

Edith Keyser White

The first African American at Rockhaven was a teacher and devoted family woman who loved travel. Edith's two daughters approached Patricia Traviss to see if she would be "willing" to accept their mother. She was initially perplexed. "The only criteria I have is if you are willing to give your mother quality care," Patricia told Friends of Rockhaven volunteers. "Why wouldn't I take her?" It had never occurred to Pat that a facility wouldn't take someone because of race. Edith came to Rockhaven because of Alzheimer's disease, but her life prior to the diagnosis is inspiring.

Born in Mobile, Alabama, in 1909, Edith Keyser came to Los Angeles at the age of ten. Edith earned a bachelor's degree in history from the University of California–Los Angeles (UCLA) and a master's degree in education from the University of Southern California (USC) in 1932. She wanted to become a teacher, but Los Angeles schools wouldn't hire her because she was black. She took a job as a social worker instead until the school system broke the color barrier in the 1940s. Edith was finally free to pursue her dream of a career in education.

She married Harry Clifton White in 1944, and the couple had three children, two daughters and a son, all of whom earned college degrees. Edith's daughters followed in their mother's footsteps by attending UCLA and entering the education field. Her son attended Yale and then Harvard Law School before returning to Los Angeles to practice law. Edith was devoted to her family and resigned from teaching in the 1950s to raise her children. In her spare time, she gardened, cooked, volunteered at the YMCA and for the Democratic Party and traveled when her children were older. In turn, her family was just as devoted to her as she had been to them. Harry dutifully cared for Edith as she began to show signs of Alzheimer's until her illness required professional assistance. Edith's life is a story of courage, determination and genuine love.

M. Louise Jung, DDS

Born in Los Angeles on April 6, 1902, M. Louise Jung was a woman far ahead of her time. She forever holds the distinction of being one of the first women to graduate from USC's dental school in the 1920s. She set up her practice in the Security Bank building in Pasadena on the corner

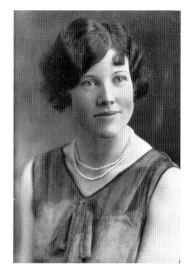

Dr. M. Louise Jung was one of the first women to graduate from USC dental school.

of Colorado and Lake. Because she never drove, she walked to work every day. In fact, exercise and healthy eating were part of a fitness routine that she maintained decades before it was fashionable.

Louise was a hands-on, do-it-yourself woman. In addition to running her own dental practice, she liked to make her own clothing and decorate her house. She repainted her home every year, and her favorite Christmas present was paint. She remained part of her Pasadena neighborhood until her retirement, when she moved to Rockhaven with her terrier, Penny. The little dog wasn't permitted to live in a cottage with Louise, but the staff at Rockhaven found a way around the problem and came up with a solution.

One of Rockhaven's nurses, Ana Taffanelli, adopted Penny and, because she lived just across the street, brought the terrier to work with her several times per week so Louise could still visit with her regularly. Louise settled into life at the Oaks Cottage, where she spent her retirement.

FRANCISZKA RADZIWON CLARK

Franciszka Radziwon was one of four children born to William, a chemical engineer, and Michalina, a housewife. She entered the world just after Christmas on December 28, 1920, in Hartford, Connecticut. After completing high school, Franciszka knew she wanted to study, so she moved to the West Coast and enrolled in UC–Berkeley. After two years of school, she moved to San Francisco in search of a job in fashion design but instead found herself working as a journalist for the *Chronicle*.

During World War II, Franciszka applied to the Women Airforce Service Pilots (WASP) in Sweetwater, Texas. She competed against 25,000 other women for a spot, and in 1942, she was one of 1,800 women accepted into the program. She was one of 1,074 women who graduated from basic training at Avenger Field. After 400 hours of ground school and 210 hours

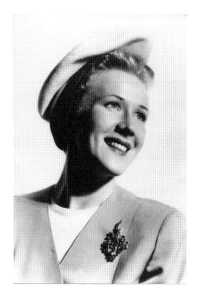

Franciszka Radziwon Clark in 1946.

of flight instruction, Franciszka piloted AT6s and AT7s at various air bases across the United States.

WASP disbanded in 1944, and soon after, Franciszka met her husband, Wallace Clark, who worked as a ski instructor in Big Bear. The couple was married for two years before divorcing, and Franciszka returned to San Francisco and the *Chronicle*, where she worked as a secretary and market analyst. She returned to Berkeley and once again set a goal to become a fashion designer. As it happened, she ended up staying in newspapers. She moved to Los Angeles, where she continued on in the newspaper business. She loved to travel and visited several places in Europe, Russia and Turkey. When she finally retired to Rockhaven, she communicated frequently with her nephews and shared her adventures of being a pilot with other residents.

NEDRA LUCRETIA SALISBURY

When Nedra Lucretia was born in Texas in 1915, she probably couldn't have imagined that her life would be filled with so much travel. But travel she did, and along the way, she carved out a life in service to others and her country.

After she attended several schools, her family moved to New Mexico, where she attended the University of New Mexico. In the 1930s, she moved to Los Angeles and completed nursing school at Los Angeles County Hospital. Because all flight attendants were required to be registered nurses in that era, Nedra went to work for United Airlines. On a flight between Burbank and San Francisco, Nedra met her future husband, Lieutenant Howard Salisbury, who was stationed at Camp Ord near Monterey. When Howard transferred to Schofield Barracks in Hawaii, she joined him, and they married in July 1941. Pearl Harbor was bombed the following December, and she was called upon to serve as a nurse at the army hospital.

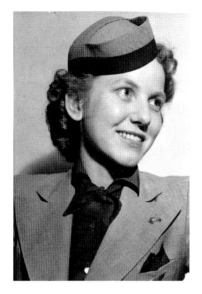

Nedra Lucretia Salisbury in her flight attendant uniform.

Not much time later, Howard and Nedra had the first of their four sons, so she and the baby fled to Los Angeles. Howard, though, continued serving in the Pacific until the war was over.

After the war, Howard continued on with the army for twenty more years. As a family, they lived for a time in war-torn Germany. Eventually, they relocated to Augusta, Georgia, before returning again to Germany, this time in Berlin, a city that was still devastated years after the war. When Howard retired, the Salisburys settled in San Francisco. They moved again, however, and lived for thirty years in Pasadena, where Nedra volunteered for the American Red Cross Disaster Program. She also worked with the South Pasadena Women's Club, the DAR and the Senior Citizens Center.

Nedra later said that she was proudest of how well her sons turned out even though they had moved so much—all four boys went to college and were successful in their chosen professions. She retired to Rockhaven, where she enjoyed walking around the gardens. All four of her sons and their families visited her regularly while she was a resident.

TAMAYE ISHIDA SHIGEMATSU

Tamaye Ishida Shigematsu was a true California girl. She was born in Los Angeles and raised near the ocean in Venice Beach. Her father had immigrated to California from Japan in 1912. He returned to Japan for his wife, and the couple settled in L.A., where Tamaye was welcomed to the world on January 6, 1922. She was the youngest of three children, with two older brothers ahead of her. Mr. Ishida started a produce trucking company, which his sons helped with as soon as they were old enough. The family also relocated from the beach to Los Angeles, where Tamaye attended Ninth Street Elementary School, Lafayette Junior High and Jefferson High School.

Tamaye discovered that, like her mother, she enjoyed sewing, and she turned out to be an excellent seamstress and dressmaker.

When the United States entered World War II after the bombing of Pearl Harbor, life took a tragic turn for the Ishida family. Because of their Japanese heritage, the family was incarcerated in May 1942 at Manzanar, located in Owens Valley. It was one of ten concentration camps in the United States for people of Japanese descent. During the war, more than 110,000 Japanese Americans were forcibly interned against their will.

It was a dark time in American history, but there was one joy that came from Tamaye's time at Manzanar. While incarcerated, she fell in love with a fellow prisoner, Joe Shigematsu, and they married in 1943. Their marriage license was issued in Lone Pine, not far from the camp, where they stayed until the war ended.

As the war ended in 1945, the couple moved to Pasadena and began the process of rebuilding their lives and creating a new one together. Joe accepted a job that meant he had to spend a few months in Philadelphia every year. Sometimes Tamaye was able to accompany him, but both of them decided this simply wasn't the life they wanted. As a couple, they started a lunch truck catering business, and it became so successful that they were able to purchase and operate a second truck.

By about 1950, they had expanded and purchased a liquor store in the Boyle Heights section of Los Angeles. Joe ran the store for seventeen years until he passed away in 1967. Tamaye carried on running the business alone for the next five years. Although she was now a widow, her life was still centered on family. Her elderly parents moved in with her so she could care for them until they, too, passed away.

Tamaye and Joe never had children of their own, but she had warm relationships with her nieces and nephews, who called her "Auntie Ta." She even put her seamstress skills to use when she made each of her nieces a wedding dress.

When Auntie Ta retired to Rockhaven, her first day was not an easy one. Now living with dementia, Tamaye was disoriented in her new surroundings. The beautiful fence surrounding Rockhaven that Agnes and Patricia took so much pride in making beautiful was troubling to Tamaye. She walked in distress around the property's perimeter next to the fence. The staff realized that Tamaye's dementia was creating confusion between Rockhaven's fence and the interment camp from decades earlier.

Tamaye eventually settled into her new home and learned she was now in a safe place. Her devoted family members continued to visit her regularly and even took her on outings to favorite Japanese restaurants or brought her to their homes for special occasions. Her entire family lived close by, so keeping that close-knit feel never changed.

Marian Witt Wexler

From an early age, quiet and polite Marian Witt displayed a talent for art. She was born in the small farming town of Beloit, Wisconsin, in 1921. In a funny coincidence, both her parents had the exact same last name—Witt—but they weren't related. To find work, Marian's father moved his family to a larger city so he could look for better employment to support the family.

As Marian grew, she was shy and sensitive but also showed a powerful streak of independence. Her artistic abilities allowed her to express herself, so after high school, she attended the Art Institute of Chicago, where she earned a scholarship. The Art Institute recognized Marian as an outstanding talent, and through the school, she was able to study in Mexico and Guatemala. Not long after, she was asked to be a full-time professor at the Art Institute. During this time, she met her husband, Haskell Wexler, with whom she made a documentary called *How to Make a Lithograph*. The Museum of Modern Art in New York later acquired the movie for its collection.

In the 1960s, Marian, Haskell and their five-year-old son, Mark, relocated to Southern California, where Haskell went on to become a prominent director of cinematography. In California, Marian formed a group of talented female artists and opened a successful gallery on Ventura Boulevard that sold their paintings, jewelry, sculpture and collages. The gallery remained open until the 1994 Northridge earthquake damaged the building.

The gallery may have closed, but it didn't stop Marian from continuing her life's work. She continued to gather like-minded artists and mentor young talent in her Malibu studio until her retirement at Rockhaven.

Anna Martin Rounds

There are a lot of things that you don't see very often. One of them is a love that lasts as long as that of Anna Martin Rounds and her husband, Edward. Anna and Edward were childhood sweethearts, and they married when she was still a teen. The marriage lasted fifty-nine years until Edward passed away.

They fell in love in Maryland, where Anna was born on October 7, 1902, in Westernport. She was the youngest of nine children. After Anna and Edward married on March 29, 1920, the couple lived at various times in Pittsburgh; Washington, D.C.; and Detroit. In 1930, they moved again, this time to Southern California. The Golden State intrigued them after they heard radio reports about the Rose Bowl and read author Zane Grey's vivid descriptions of the desert. As soon as they arrived, they knew they had made the right decision. Although they visited friends and family in Maryland, California was now home.

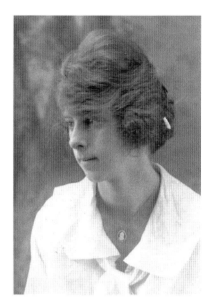

Anna Martin Rounds in 1918.

They made their home in L.A.'s Echo Park neighborhood, where they had their only child, a daughter named Rayma, who was born in 1932. They moved up north for a while to San Francisco but returned to Los Angeles in 1957. Rayma, meanwhile, attended college, majoring in geography at San Francisco State College and then receiving a master's in library science from USC, where she went on to become a librarian. She also later worked at Occidental College and the California Institute of Technology in Pasadena.

Anna spent her retirement gardening and loved the outdoors, including watching wildlife and birds. Anna and Edward drove all over the United States sightseeing and covered ground from the West all the way to Niagara Falls. Edward passed away in 1979, after the couple had spent a lifetime together. Anna maintained their home in Whittier for a while before retiring to Rockhaven.

BERNICE ZURBACH

In an era when many women had few options, Bernice Zurbach dedicated her life to education and furthering women's causes. Originally from

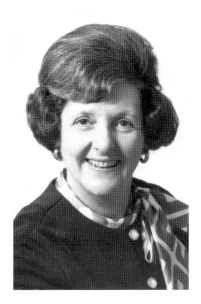

Bernice Zurback in 1971.

Spokane, Washington, Bernice earned a bachelor's, master's and PhD from the University of Washington. She and her husband, Robert, moved to Pasadena and raised their two kids, a son named Randy and a daughter, Christine.

During her lifetime, Bernice served as a delegate for the United Nations Decade for Women, attending the 1975 conference in Mexico City. She also attended the mid-decade event in Copenhagen in 1980 and the closing conference in Nairobi, Kenya, in 1985. She was a member of the California Conference Organizing Committee for the International Women's Year Conference in Los Angeles in 1977 and a delegate to the United States International Women's Year Conference in 1978. She retired to Rockhaven and passed away in September 1988 of lung ailments.

BETTY JANE FAIRLEY

Although she was born and raised in California, Betty Jane Fairley's parents were immigrants from Scotland. It goes without saying that during her lifetime, Betty Jane enjoyed the Scottish games, dances and other traditional Scottish presentations.

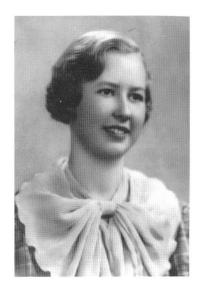

Betty Jane Fairley was a teacher and the first female bus driver for the Los Angeles School District. She also worked as a governess for Ronald and Nancy Reagan's children.

As a young woman, Betty Jane worked as a teacher and became the first female bus driver in the Los Angeles School District. She also worked for a while as a governess to Ronald and Nancy Reagan's children.

She traveled the world—all over the United States, Europe, Scandinavia and even the Arctic Circle. She lived in Pasadena and participated in the Shakespeare Club and community service projects. After a life of caring for children and globetrotting, Betty Jane retired to Rockhaven.

EDITH VAN BUREN

Edith Van Buren's family had deep roots in Bavaria, where they were from. Edith herself was born and raised in Munich, where she studied commerce and literature. She loved reading, playing the piano, dancing and music. It's likely she would have stayed in her hometown forever, but World War II disrupted the lives of citizens all over Germany, Edith included. In December 1938, at the age of thirty, Edith and her husband made their way to safety in Zurich, Switzerland. From there, they traveled to Holland and then finally boarded a transatlantic ship bound for the United States.

Once on American soil, Edith and her husband met up with her brother, who had arrived two years prior. In honor of his new country, he served in the United States Army during the war. Soon, her parents also made their way to the United States, and the entire family was reunited. In 1944, as the war still raged on, Edith became an American citizen in a Los Angeles courtroom. She settled into her new life and lived in various states, including New Mexico and Hawaii, and in Palm Springs, California. At one point, she owned her own restaurant and worked as a bookstore manager and at a resort hotel. After a life so full of experience, travel and war, Edith retired to a quiet life at Rockhaven.

DOROTHY GEORGE SPRINGER

Dorothy George was a Chicago native born on March 12, 1899, but she lived in several cities and traveled the globe in adulthood. She came west to attend college, first at Stanford University in Northern California and then south to earn a master's at USC in social work. Upon completing her education, she headed off to New York and lived in Greenwich Village while attending the prestigious Parsons School of Design. She later took a job in the Works Project Administration (WPA), a Roosevelt administration program set up to help provide jobs during the Great Depression.

As a photographer, Dorothy made a pictorial history of the Pit River Indians of Northern California, a band known for fine basketry work. Her photographs and old glass plates were donated to the Southwest Museum in Los Angeles, which houses one of the best collections of Native American artifacts in the West.

Dorothy finally settled in Los Angeles, where she lived with her husband, Norman Springer, a screenwriter and author. Their home overlooked Elysian Park and was built by one of Frank Lloyd Wright's disciples. Dorothy and Norman filled their home with artifacts

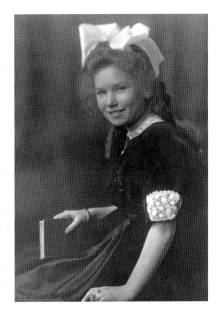

Dorothy Springer as she appeared in childhood.

they collected from their world travels, which included China, Indonesia, Australia, New Zealand, Alaska, Mexico, New Guinea and Europe.

Dorothy took steps to ensure that others who were passionate about art and travel would have similar opportunities. She gave back by becoming a patron of the Sierra Club, the Pacific Asia Museum, the Los Angeles Museum of Art and the Los Angeles Symphony.

While at Rockhaven, Dorothy liked to recall her adventures in the desert and the Angeles National Forest. Traveling to such locations was hazardous in the days before there were highways, but as a devoted nature lover and conservationist, she was never deterred.

Chapter 8
Rockhaven Closes

Since she took over Rockhaven from her grandmother, Agnes Richards, in the 1960s, the property had continued to prosper under the leadership of Patricia Traviss. The residents of Rockhaven enjoyed a safe, peaceful life surrounded by lush gardens, caring employees and activities to keep their minds and bodies active. By 2001, though, Patricia was ready to retire. Rockhaven as a business and the property itself were sold to Ararat Home Los Angeles Inc., another local and respected elder-care company.

Like Rockhaven, Ararat had a reputation for high-quality care. Founded in 1949 in Los Angeles, Ararat was originally created to meet the needs of the local Armenian community. Over the years, Ararat was so successful that it began expanding its business to other campuses in the Greater Los Angeles area to accommodate growth.

Life at Rockhaven continued on under Ararat's supervision, but it became clear that things would run differently now that it was owned by a corporation. Ararat maintained adequate care standards, but the special touches that Agnes Richards had put in place, and then were carried on by her granddaughter Patricia Traviss, ceased. The monthly newsletters that kept family members informed fell by the wayside. The Easter and Mother's Day teas were called off, as were the holiday celebrations and Sunday night dinners for visiting family members. The once-lush gardens and rose bushes Ivan Cole had prided himself on were no longer award-winning quality.

Soon after Ararat took over, it became apparent that the grounds needed updating. The facility had always been well maintained, but with

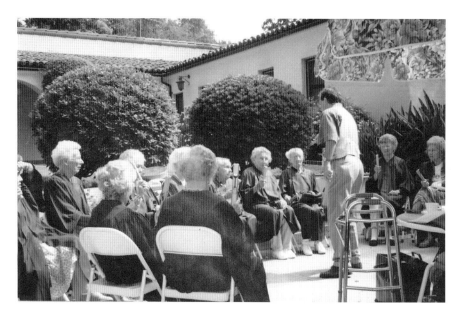

Rockhaven prided itself on keeping the residents busy, which helped their brains stay active. Oftentimes this helped their illnesses from getting worse. Here, a guest conductor leads a group of women with dementia in a bell recital.

several buildings dating back to the 1920s or before, routine maintenance could easily get expensive. Furthermore, ADA regulations had changed considerably over the years, and Rockhaven's grounds needed to modernize and meet new standards. Ararat decided the property wasn't worth the financial investments needed to keep it open. Although it was purchased in 2001, Ararat shuttered Rockhaven just five years later in 2006.

The closure of a local landmark created quite a stir when it hit the newspapers. In addition to the property closing, the staff would soon be out of work, and worse, dozens of elderly women had nowhere to go. Many of the ladies had lived comfortably at Rockhaven for years, and now families were looking to find suitable new accommodations for their wives, mothers and grandmothers. The trauma this caused the elderly women, many of whom suffered from Alzheimer's or dementia, triggered outrage among the family members.

Rockhaven's profit margins weren't high enough to meet Ararat's expectations, so plans were announced to level the 1923-era property and replace it with a large-scale elder-care facility. Locals quickly objected to the massive development plan. Concern grew over the property itself, as well as twenty-six California oak trees that remained

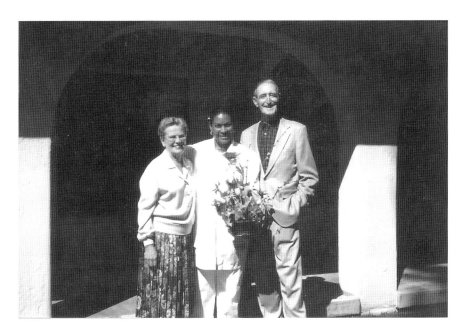

Gardener and horticulturist Ivan Cole was one of the few full-time male employees during Rockhaven's history. Here he poses for a picture with some female staff members. When the property was threatened with demolition, Ivan came out of retirement to speak on behalf of Rockhaven's legacy and importance to the community.

on the five-acre property, which were historical in and of themselves. When one oak tree had to be removed in the early 1960s because of root rot, it was determined that it was approximately six hundred years old. Horticulturist Ivan Cole, then eighty-seven and retired since 1997, was heartbroken and quoted in a local newspaper as saying, "The oaks are the only thing we can save."

Ararat's chairman of the board, John Yalbezian, didn't comment on Rockhaven's status publicly but announced in August 2006 that the company would sell the property "as is" instead of razing it. When it was put on the market, however, Ararat's For Sale sign advertised the property divided into eleven lots. Locals feared that a developer would indeed buy the land and cut it up. Questions began to arise about what would become of the now-historic property that had served the community for generations. Because Ararat wouldn't comment, it only fueled rumors. Mike Lawler, president of the Historical Society of the Crescenta Valley, was quoted in the local newspaper as saying that closing Rockhaven was a betrayal to the community and to the residents who had lived there.

For two years, the property sat empty. In April 2008, the City of Glendale finally stepped in and purchased the property for $8.25 million. The city planned to preserve the property and repurpose the grounds and buildings for a park, community center and public library.

The city promptly began assessing the property for preservation, with fourteen of its fifteen buildings under serious consideration for landmarking. The city also hired twenty-four-hour security to watch the grounds and began restoring the caretaker's cottage.

Locals were thrilled to hear this news. When plans were announced in 2008, more than one hundred residents showed up at the June meeting for the Historical Society of the Crescenta Valley to discuss Rockhaven's future. Also discussed was the newly formed volunteer group to maintain the property and keep it clean. Guest speakers that night included Ivan Cole, who fondly recalled his days at Rockhaven and Agnes Richards, and Jay Platt, the historic preservation planner for Glendale.

That same month, June 2008, the city hired Valley Crest Landscape Management for debris removal and landscaping. The estimated cost was $48,125 for site cleanup, shrub removal and trimming. But just as people got their hopes up for the rebirth of Rockhaven, misfortune struck, and the economy crashed in the fall of 2008. Any money that would have gone toward preserving Rockhaven was now diverted to other places. Once again, Rockhaven would have to sit empty for the foreseeable future.

Rockhaven remained abandoned for the next seven years, save the occasional volunteer sweeping the grounds to keep them clear of debris. During those years, the City of Glendale went through changes, which included new priorities and different city council members. When Glendale was finally ready to revisit Rockhaven in 2015, prospective plans were vastly different than they had been in 2008.

The new city council didn't have the same enthusiasm for Rockhaven that the previous council had. Besides, after the economic recession they were also looking for ideas that could bring revenue into the city, as opposed to a park or library. The maintenance of Rockhaven was costing Glendale $50,000 annually even though it was abandoned. It didn't take long for the city council to determine that selling or leasing the languishing property to developers was a viable option. When word got back to the community, people were more than disappointed. They were furious.

Rockhaven had been part of the community for more than ninety years. It had become more than just a sanitarium. It was a symbol of progressive mental healthcare and treatment. It was a feminist landmark. There was

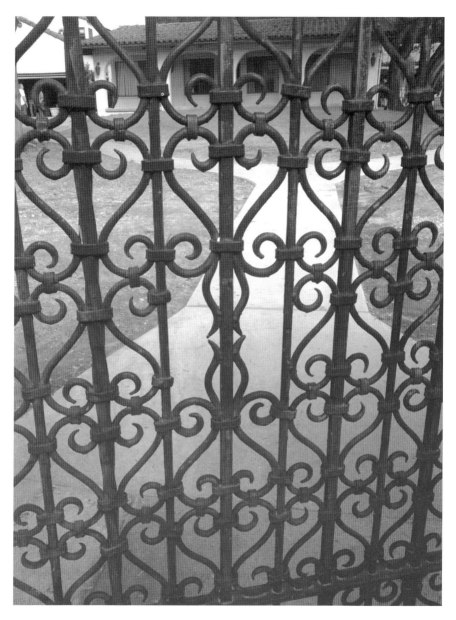

Rockhaven currently sits empty as a nonprofit group, the Friends of Rockhaven, works to save the property and respectfully repurpose the buildings with developers. Everything currently remains intact, and the fine details of the past are still visible, such as the elegant wrought ironwork.

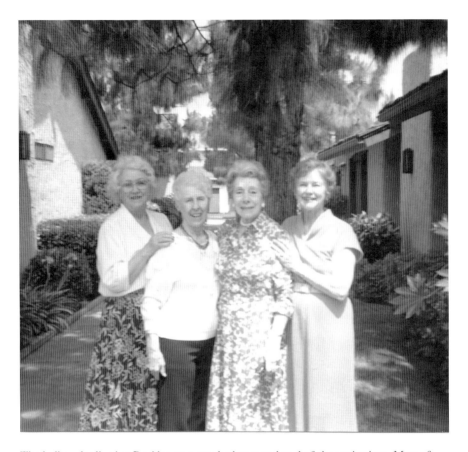

The ladies who lived at Rockhaven were the heart and soul of the sanitarium. Most of them thrived in the environment and were either able to go home after an illness or live out their days in peace. As psychiatric treatment changed in the 1960s with prescription drugs and better therapy, Rockhaven became more of a rest home for dementia patients and retirement.

Hollywood history attached to the facility. It was a one-of-a-kind sociological achievement. In short, Rockhaven had become a genuine cultural landmark since it first opened in 1923.

Agnes Richards had fought hard during her lifetime to protect Rockhaven. Now volunteers and local residents were ready to take up the cause again to protect the legacy she made. The Friends of Rockhaven, a nonprofit group of volunteers, stepped up and began looking in earnest for opportunities to save the property. Efforts included running tours of the three-and-a-half-acre campus, which was left perfectly intact after residents and staff vacated. For the first time, community members, neighbors and history buffs were given the opportunity to see the unique property in person and behind the scenes. Being able to actually walk through the bungalows, hospital area, dining room and gardens enabled visitors to experience the space rather than just hearing or reading about it. Because the property was not technically open to the public, tours were free of charge. At the end of the tours, however, guests were given the opportunity to become members of the Friends of Rockhaven and strengthen the organization. Fundraisers were held, and Joanna Linkchorst, the Friends of Rockhaven's president, tirelessly spoke to groups and at city council meetings to save the property.

The year 2016 turned out to have some positive movement forward for saving Rockhaven. Under the direction of Joanna, the nonprofit was able to place Rockhaven in both the California and National Registers of Historic Places. In April, the State Historical Resources Commission unanimously agreed to the designation during a meeting in San Francisco. Friends of Rockhaven had sought the help of the Historical Resources Group, a historical preservation organization in Pasadena, to help get Rockhaven nominated. The nomination and approval included the buildings, gardens and historic oak trees that dotted the landscape.

There were several ideas for what would become of Rockhaven, including turning it back into a health facility. Joanna, however, was determined to keep the property available to the public so everyone could visit. "We're really hoping that something more historically geared will come from this," she told the *Los Angeles Times*. "I want [the buildings] to be alive with art and commerce and food."

Once the state designation was in place, Rockhaven was eligible to proceed on to a national nomination. Not everyone in Glendale was happy about Rockhaven's official historic status. City Manager Scott Ochoa had written a letter in February to Julianne Polanco, the historic preservation officer for California. In it, he said the city was concerned that a historic status might deter developers from working with the property. The city was hoping for a historical designation, he said, *after* the property had been redeveloped.

"Our decision not to support the pending National Register nomination reflects only our concern that some developers may be—needlessly, we recognize—apprehensive about buying a listed property," his letter said. Despite his objections, Rockhaven's nomination was approved.

Later in the year, Glendale City Council began listening to proposals from seven development firms. After hearing the presentations, a selection committee met to determine Rockhaven's fate. The committee ranked the proposals by six criteria: preservation dedication, open space and

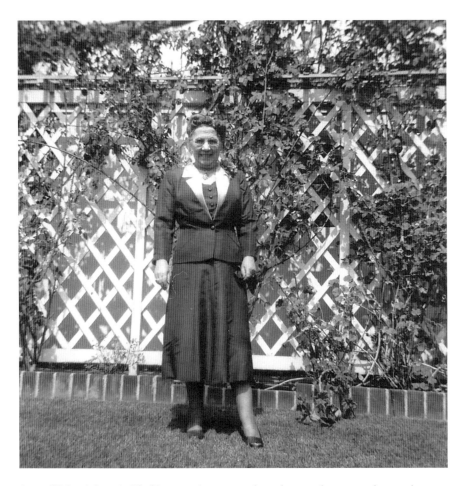

Agnes Richards later in life. She started as a nurse in asylums and progressed to owning a private sanitarium that prided itself on putting the residents first. Today, a group of volunteers maintains her property and works to preserve its history.

accessibility, developer experience, neighborhood compatibility, return on investment and use for community groups.

Among the proposals were a plan for a forty-five-room hotel, building houses on the land for first-time home buyers and turning the property back into a mental health hospital setting. In the end, a proposal by Gangi Design LED Build was selected. Gangi's design turned the land into park space and the buildings into boutique retail spaces. There would also be space for nonprofits and a Crescenta Valley Museum. Glendale mayor Paula Devine said selecting a proposal hadn't been an easy decision and that community

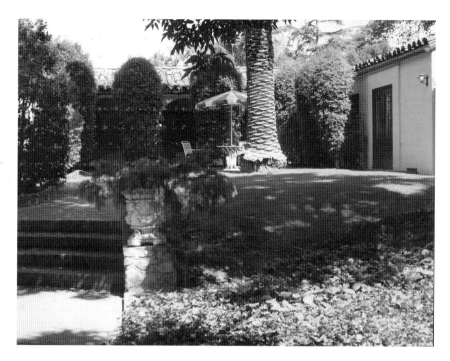

Rockhaven remains intact, though it is currently unoccupied. The question remains of what to do with this historically significant property. Friends of Rockhaven president Joanna Linkchorst would like to see part of the property turned into a museum and other buildings into boutique retail spaces.

feedback played an important factor. "I selected Gangi for an important reason, mainly because it satisfies my goals for Rockhaven and, more importantly, the desires of the majority of our community," she said in a *Los Angeles Times* article. "I feel that Rockhaven is a jewel in our community…so I really feel that the city needs to retain ownership of this property."

After some discussion, the city council voted unanimously for the boutique commercial center and park plan. In that same *Los Angeles Times* article, developer Matt Gangi said, "We didn't know what to expect, but we're excited about it, to turn [Rockhaven] into an activated park space and cultural site."

As Rockhaven gets ready to enter its next phase, optimism remains high that it will be reborn as a cultural hub that serves the community as it always has—just in a new way.

Bibliography

Newspapers

Akron Beacon Journal. "Babe Egan Is Palace Star." February 13, 1929.

Anderson, Tre'vell. "Where Time Is Frozen." *Los Angeles Times*, August 16, 2015.

Arizona Republic. "Actress' Mother Is Found Dead." October 20, 1938.

Arnold, Marion. "Producers Who Happen to See Winnemucca Boy Dance Start Him on Road to Success." *Nevada State Journal*, December 13, 1931.

Asheville Citizen-Times. "Gable Marries Widow of Douglas Fairbanks." December 21, 1949.

Bingham, Hilda. "Women and Events: Gwen Lee." *Pensacola News Journal*, December 13, 1925.

Casper Star-Tribune. "Hollywood Redheads to Open Engagement at Rialto Saturday." April 16, 1926.

Chicago Tribune. "Cummins' Band Leads Show in Empire Room." February 27, 1938.

———. "Drops Suit to Name Guardian for Gwen Lee." April 2, 1932.

———. "Richman Stays at Chez Paree Until April 10." March 27, 1938.

———. "Suzy Says." November 19, 1970.

Columbus (NE) Journal, January 5, 1910.

Cooper, Charles. "City Buys Rockhaven." *Valley Sun*, March 21, 2008.

———. "Rockhaven Purchase Completed." *Valley Sun*, April 11, 2008.

Corrigan, Kelly. "Glendale Objected to Historical Designation for Rockhaven Site." *Los Angeles Times*, May 3, 2016.

Courier-News. "Hollywood's Twelve Most Beautiful Girls." July 17, 1924.

Cumberland (MD) Sunday Times. March 25, 1951.

Daily Journal (Vineland, NJ). "Babe Egan First Girl Band Leader." December 3, 1934.

Daily Review (Decatur, Illinois). "Clark Gable's Ex-Wife Will Be Drama Teacher." December 27, 1939.

Des Moines Register. "Mrs. Gable No. 1 Had Talk with the No. 2." December 27, 1939.

Diamond, Robert S. "Mary Florence (Babe) Egan: Another Hollywood Star of 1920s Dies." *Los Angeles Times*, February 9, 1966.

Dixon, Hugh. "Hollywood." *Pittsburgh Post-Gazette*, February 7, 1944.

Edwardsville (IL) Intelligencer. "Gable Spurns Reconciliation Try." June 1, 1950.

Eureka Humboldt Standard (UPI). "MM's Mother Found Hiding." July 6, 1963.

Gallegos, Bianca P. "Rockhaven to Be Sold?" *Los Angeles Times*, August 25, 2006.

Gilchrist, Tracy E. "Oak Trees Hang in Balance." *Los Angeles Times*, September 23, 2016.

Goldworthy, Robin. "Armchair 'Tour' of Rockhaven." *Los Angeles Times*, June 6, 2008.

Graham, Sheila. "Hollywood Today." *Star Press* (Muncie, IN), May 28, 1939.

————. "Sylvia Stanley Gable Has a Lucky Star!" *Pittsburgh Post-Gazette*, January 16, 1950.

Harrison, Paul. "In Hollywood." *Ironwood (MI) Daily Globe*, March 7, 1939.

Honolulu Star-Bulletin. "Babe Egan's 'Hollywood Redheads.'" December 15, 1925.

Kearney (NE) Daily Hub. "Young Lepinski Ends Life." April 17, 1911.

Kester, Marshall. "Guests Dress Up." *Los Angeles Times*, June 7, 1936.

Kingsley, Grace. "Modern Romance Viewed; Cinema Gossip Related." *Los Angeles Times*, January 12, 1934.

Lawler, Mike. "Spike Jones Market." *Crescenta Valley Weekly*, August 16, 2011.

Lincoln Star. "Many New and Youthful Stars Appearing on Silver Screen in Answer to Public's Demands." November 22, 1925.

Los Angeles Times. "Cloak and Suit House Action Names Gwen Lee." October 17, 1932.

————. "Conservator Named for Miss Monroe's Mother." December 3, 1959.

————. "Ern Westmore Weds Actress." February 16, 1941.

————. "Exposition's Finale Will Be Tonight." October 20, 1925.

———. "Gable's Fifth Wife Kay Left All of His Estate." November 24, 1960.

———. "Given at Beach." September 20, 1925.

———. "Hollywood Beauties Form Culture Club." September 16, 1923.

———. "Mrs. Fairbanks's Sister Arrives." April 18, 1937.

———. "Peggy Fears' Mother Found Dead from Gas" October 20, 1938.

———. "Peggy Fears; Ziegfeld Follies Showgirl (Obituary)." August 27, 1994.

———. "U.S. Jury Indicts Six on Income Tax Charges." February 12, 1959.

———. "Widow Fined $9,000 for Tax Evasion." November 17, 1959.

L.U.K. "What to Do, What to See." *Harrisburg Telegraph*, November 30, 1934.

Moffitt, John C. "Billy Gable Married Josephine Dillon." *Des Moines Tribune*, October 20, 1932.

———. "The Climb of Clark Gable." *Atlanta Constitution*, October 23, 1932.

Montana Standard. "Former Resident Dies in Seattle." August 8, 1943.

Nebraska State Journal. April 16, 1911

———. "Fire at Hastings." August 6, 1910.

———. "Gwen Lee Called Back." July 19, 1931.

News-Messenger (Fremont, OH). "Peggy Fears Find the Way." September 2, 1960.

Oakland (CA) Tribune. December 29, 1944.

———. "Mother Sues Film Actress." March 11, 1932.

Palm Beach Post. "Big Crowd Throngs Auditorium to Witness Annual Dance Revue of Irene Lake Studio Last Night." April 18, 1935.

Playfair, Polly. "Peggy Fears and 'Blumey' Are Back Together Again—Which Shows What Love Can Do in Turning an Amazing Agreement to Disagree into a Scrap of Paper." *Salt Lake Tribune*, July 30, 1939.

Post-Standard. "Film Star's Heirs Notified: Taxes Eat Up Marilyn's Million Dollars." June 22, 1966.

Rhinelander Daily News (Associated Press). "Mother Asks to Be Star's Conservator." November 6, 1959.

Rogers, Adela. "The Gable I Knew: The Woman Who Molded a King." *St. Johns Philadelphia Daily News*, November 25, 1960.

Santa Ana Register. "Return to Vaudeville." February 28, 1925.

Shaffer, George. "Will James to Get 3-Way Play in Films." *Chicago Tribune*, March 14, 1932.

Shearer, Lloyd. "Clark Gable: After 25 Years in Hollywood, He's on His Own." *Independent Press-Telegram* (Long Beach, CA), June 19, 1955.

Shreveport Times. "Good Neighbors." August 11, 1942.

Smith, Liz. Media Meow. *Valley News* (Van Nuys, CA), September 18, 1977.

Stein, Edwin C. "Former 'Follies' Star Now Stage's Youngest Producer." *Pittsburgh Post-Gazette*, March 19, 1932.

Tennessean. "Gwen Lee Signs with Metro-Goldwyn-Mayer." August 16, 1925.

Van Nuys News. "This Week in 1928." August 4, 1938.

Weinstock, Bob. "A Scottsdale Woman Remembers Beating the Drums for the Hollywood Redheads." *Arizona Republic*, February 17, 1974.

Wilkes-Barre Times Leader. "At Poli's." May 10, 1927.

Wilson, Earl. "Even in Death Trouble Dogs Marilyn." *Miami News*, June 21, 1965.

———. "Marilyn Monroe Story Takes a Sadder Twist." *Lansing State Journal*, September 15, 1966.

———. "Marilyn's Mother Unaware of Sad Estate News." *Bristol Daily Courier*, July 1, 1965.

Books

Bly, Nellie. *Ten Days in a Mad-House*. N.p., 2015 (original publication 1887).

Finnegan, W. Robert. *The Barlow Story*. San Bernardino, CA: Crown Printers, 1992.

Goessel, Tracey. *The First King of Hollywood: The Life of Douglas Fairbanks*. Chicago: Chicago Review Press, 2016.

Goffman, Irving. *Asylums*. New York: Anchor Books, 1961.

Harris, Warren G. *Clark Gable: A Biography*. New York: Crown Publishing Group, 2002.

Hayter-Menzies. *Mrs. Ziegfeld*. Jefferson, NC: McFarland & Co., 2009.

Lawler, Mike. *Crescenta Valley History Hidden in Plain Sight*. Charleston, SC: Arcadia Publishing, 2017.

Lawler, Mike, and Robert Newcombe. Images of America: *La Crescenta*. Charleston, SC: Arcadia Publishing, 2005.

Lawler, Mike, and Robert Newcombe with the Historical Society of the Crescenta Valley. Then & Now: *The Crescenta Valley*. Charleston, SC: Arcadia Publishing, 2010.

Newcombe, Robert. *Montrose*. Charleston, SC: Arcadia Publishing, 2013.

Websites

Ancestry.com.

Fire Island Pines Historical Preservation Society. "Pines People—Peggy Fears." www.pineshistory.org/fires-and-storms/the-peggy-fears-story-part-1.

Library of Congress. "Stadler, Marion, 1912–." id.loc.gov/authorities/names/nr96018748.html.

Index

About the Author

Elisa Jordan is a freelance writer and editor who specializes in history, architecture and pets. When not writing, she is working to promote tourism in Southern California and giving tours in Los Angeles. She is the founder of L.A. Woman Tours and considered an authority on several aspects of Los Angeles history, including Marilyn Monroe, The Doors and the Hollywood music scene. Elisa is a native Californian whose family dates back to about 1915 in the state.

Visit us at
www.historypress.com
....